Chronic LOVE

Trusting God While Suffering with A Chronic Illness

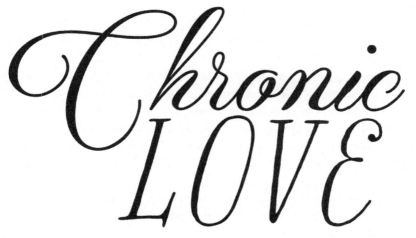

Chronic LOVE

Trusting God While Suffering with A Chronic Illness

BROOKE BARTZ

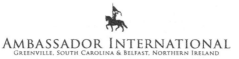

Ambassador International
GREENVILLE, SOUTH CAROLINA & BELFAST, NORTHERN IRELAND

www.ambassador-international.com

Chronic Love

Trusting God While Suffering with A Chronic Illness

© 2019 by Brooke Bartz

All rights reserved

ISBN: 978-1-62020-924-0
eISBN: 978-1-62020-939-4
Library of Congress Control Number: 2019935296

Unless otherwise marked, Scripture taken from the NEW AMERICAN STANDARD BIBLE®, Copyright ©1960,1962,1963,1968,1971,1972,1973,1975,197 7,1995 by The Lockman Foundation. Used by permission.

Scripture marked ESV taken from The Holy Bible, English Standard Version. ESV® Text Edition: 2016. Copyright ©2001 by Crossway Bibles, a publishing ministry of Good News Publishers.

Cover Design & Typesetting by Hannah Nichols
Edited by Daphne Self

AMBASSADOR INTERNATIONAL
Emerald House
411 University Ridge, Suite B14
Greenville, SC 29601, USA
www.ambassador-international.com

AMBASSADOR BOOKS
The Mount
2 Woodstock Link
Belfast, BT6 8DD, Northern Ireland, UK
www.ambassadormedia.co.uk

The colophon is a trademark of Ambassador, a Christian publishing company.

Dedicated to my husband,
My soul mate, the man of God's choosing, who continues to see that
I am saturated daily in the balm of God's word. You love me as Jesus
Christ calls the husband to lay down his life. Life with you is richer,
fuller, lovelier, it is Christ like, and real and oh so deep. You have
taught me to breathe in as my exhausted diaphragm expands to take
in each breath that God gives me and exhale praising the Lord joy-
fully. Whatever the day holds and the future tomorrows, I will love
you with every fiber of my being.

To my daughter,
I am so thankful for the gift of you, and that God chose me to be
your mommy. I love you more than sprinkles on cupcakes! You are
my quirky, compassionate, beautiful, bright ball of sunshine. May
the Lord call your name, and may your greatest heart's cry and
prayer be, "Thy kingdom come Thy will be done on earth as it is in
Heaven." Let your life be used as a torch and flame to light the way
for those in the blindness of sin's hold.

To Penny Amack,
You are my treasured friend and ever faithful spiritual sister and
mentor. Your wisdom and council give me strength to see this trial
as an opportunity to put the love of Christ on display. I am thankful
beyond words for God's providence and how He picked you out to
disciple and grow me as a Proverbs 31 woman. I love you!

Dedicated to the memory of Sue Wyatt,
My forever sister in Christ who endured a chronic disease and fought
the good fight. Her life I hold close to my heart knowing the promise

of a perfected body one day. She helped pave the way for me to walk this trial. Her faith and trust in the Savior I pray resonate in my life. To someone whose shoes should never be filled. I love you and I will See you in Glory!

To my mother,
Who continues to endure Multiple sclerosis. May you know the Great Physician's peace. Thank you for being my mom and being with me on this journey. You will always have my forever love and utmost devotion.

To all my bosom sisters,
Thank you for being so faithful to be the hands and feet of Christ and to give so much in selfless love. Every day I wake up praising God for each one of you. You are each a spiritual backbone that continues to prop me up against the cross. Your self-sacrificing hearts are what the early church did as they served the body of Christ. You have given meals, time, love, encouragement, performed acts of kindness, laughed with me, cried with me, held me accountable, loved my daughter as your own, and have been my prayer warriors and stood with me as I continue to fight this disease. I love you all!

To Karen Steinmann,
Not only my amazing editor but my sister and dear friend in Jesus Christ. Thank you for everything and inspiring me to press on because of the impact your son Luke's life made on me. He would be so proud of you! Till you see him in Heaven and I finally get to meet him there! I look forward to that day when there is no more pain or weeping.

CONTENTS

FOREWORD

Dear Reader,

It is my privilege to write the foreword on this book, as I know the author very well, and have witnessed the physical battle she endures everyday, every moment of her life since her diagnosis. I have watched her move from learning to cope and deal with such a pervasive and yet elusive disease, to treatment along with all the side effects of meds that presume to help, into a young woman who by God's grace has embraced this disease to His glory. Brooke has used her pain-wrought days and nights to invest in heavenly benefits for herself, for any who battle chronic diseases, have incurred devastating losses, and for those who walk these difficult paths with those they love.

In this her first book, you will find answers to questions, reasons, and results for why one suffers, as well as how to manage and cope with said sufferings from many perspectives, (as the sufferer, the care-giver, or one who watches from the sidelines). Brooke lays out in detail the attitude and perspective one can have when each of us surrenders to the love and saving grace of the Lord Jesus and God of heaven.

I will re-read and reference this book for encouragement in my own life, and to encourage others whose path is wrought with affliction, turmoil, pain and suffering, no matter the type, source, struggle or perspective. For in it, Brooke gives reason and even rationale for the assault, then offers the reader the strength and the support needed to cope with and even rest in the battle, with the Lord's guidance and counsel . . . from His Word.

This little book is filled with references, even quotes that are relevant to every "help" she offers, and since it comes first hand, from one who has and continues to walk an increasingly debilitating disease, she speaks from a position of authority.

Keep this book readily available in your library, keep an extra on hand to give away, and refer often to the Bible, as it is the book wherein Brooke derives her focus, strength, peace, and abiding faith in her Lord.

—Penny Amack

Chapter One

A CHRONIC JOURNEY

"Our sufferings may be lasting, not everlasting."
– Thomas Watson

In this you greatly rejoice, even though now for a little while, if necessary, you have been distressed by various trials, so that the proof of your faith, being more precious than gold which is perishable, even though tested by fire, may be found to result in praise and glory and honor at the revelation of Jesus Christ.
– 1 Peter 1:6-7

To My New Friends,

In the following pages, you'll discover an open book of carefully chosen words, penned in the quiet nooks of my heart's journal and now, putting pen to paper, offered as hope-filled letters to you. If you're a woman with a disease or disability, or if you're a caregiver of one with disease, please know you're not alone. This book is a beating testimony and burden of sheer love and devotion, borne of a profound desire to write and speak to your surrendered soul and spur you on in your own chronic journey with this deeply trying, often complex, but effectually wincing affliction.

The disease or disability you're enduring is God's chosen will for you, and it may be gone tomorrow, or you may carry it with you for the rest of your life. I find comfort in the apostle Paul's divinely-inspired words, "... *in everything give thanks; for this is God's will for you in Christ Jesus*" (1 Thessalonians 5:18). Like me, your life may be enmeshed with disease or disability—but your life doesn't abound in it. If you're a believer in our Lord, Jesus Christ, then experiencing a disease doesn't ever change the fact that you're an heir to the King and kept by the merciful and consuming affection of a Father who cares for you. He doesn't turn His head in disgust or ignorance or dismiss your disease and the trials you face; but He has ordained it.

... who has saved us and called us with a holy calling, not according to our works, but according to His own purpose and grace which was granted us in Christ Jesus from all eternity.
– 2 Timothy 1:9

Your affliction doesn't make you who you are or limit what you can do in God's eyes and expectations. Limitations comprise the world's definition of a chronic disease or disability; but this definition illuminates culture's folly. Know deep in your soul, my new friend, that you are loved. You are a daughter of the Lord of lords.

For we are His workmanship, created in Christ Jesus for good works, which God prepared beforehand so that we would walk in them.
– Ephesians 2:10

Being a believer makes you different. You are on a spiritual conquest to tell of Christ's gift of salvation by speaking and sharing the Gospel and by leading with one intent and purpose of making His name known. You make His name known by communicating the Gospel and by living as a testimony through the work of salvation that Christ has done in your life.

The greatest adventure in this life is living for Christ. Just as Paul understood that being on this earth means fruitful life for Christ, he also knew that departing the earth to live in Heaven meant no more pain and an eternity in the presence of his soul's Creator face-to-face. When God chose to leave Paul on this earth, He knew Paul's ministry was not complete. In the same way, even though you bear disease or disability, God has you on this earth because your life, your great adventure, your ceaseless journey, is not yet finished; your ministry is not complete. Your life exudes His purpose and meaning; you are the Lord's. Look at what Paul says speaking to the church at Philippi to give them, and us, faith and strength:

> *For to me, to live is Christ and to die is gain. But if I am to live on in the flesh, this* will mean *fruitful labor for me; and I do not know which to choose. But I am hard-pressed from both* directions, *having the desire to depart and be with Christ, for that is very much better; yet to remain on in the flesh is more necessary for your sake.*
>
> – Philippians 1:21-24

I pray that the desire to live for Christ will bubble up in your soul for the sake of the Gospel. As we suffer, may we seek out living for Christ in passionate devotion to His saving grace. May we echo Paul's voice, even with our perilous, hard-pressed trial.

DEDICATED TO YOU

This book is for you, my precious sister. Not only have I written this for those experiencing a recurrent disease, syndrome, or disability, but this book is also for the caregiver who walks with and beside you, selflessly striving to uplift the brunt of your peril as you suffer in the providential hand of hardship.

This book is for the unbeliever, the one in hardened disbelief of the God who created her. It's for the person turning to the false gods that always let us down—to the placebos that trick and belittle the Truth and offer only spiritual death. This book is for the believer who knows the sinless Savior but is fighting to find joy and contentment despite the cruelty of disease. This is for the woman contending with the destruction of cancer, trying every experimental drug and praying she will be healed. It's for the wife feeling helpless as the effects of her husband's disease have brought a financial burden as he can no longer work outside the home. This book is also for the mom sitting at her child's hospital bedside, watching the monitor, waiting on the doctor, and begging God for a new prognosis. It's for the teenage girl unable to walk and now using a wheelchair instead of her own legs. This is for the woman who daily becomes sicker and feebler, trying to navigate unchartered waters and trials pressed upon her, seeking to remain brave in faith but feeling alone in solitude and losing ground. It's for every woman who feels tired and worn, holding onto life like the climber braving a mountain with blistered hands, losing her grip on the frayed rope that secures her steps.

This book, I pray, reaches the permanently disabled woman or teenage girl; I pray it finds its way before the eyes of the young lady just diagnosed with a terminal illness, desperately needing assurance—to be held up, loved, and hugged—as she starts the fight of her life. This is for the missionary overseas looking into both the young and old faces of sickness and death. It's for the parents who just said goodbye to a life well nurtured, their adored fairing, the given now cradled in eternity, now timelessly wrapped in God's nurturing arms. Faced with this unspeakable loss, the child's mother—now finding herself lost in despair and misery, unable to see the cross on the hill and grieving without the understanding of a sovereign God—now needs hope and needs the Savior.

Losses like these of insurmountable depth cause paralyzing shock and solemn silence—the silence of being without, a silence louder than a piercing siren, and one you never want to hear again. Have you experienced loss, the kind that makes you miss someone so much that the pain buffets your soul? Have you experienced memories that keep assailing you when you hear a familiar sound, inhale a favorite scent, or pass by someone who resembles your loved one now gone? These kinds of photographic images move like an icy breeze that brings in the unwelcome season of winter recollections amidst the questions and grief of all the "whys" left unanswered. And, even though we try to understand God's plan and seek the purpose in the pain, the anguish of soft snowflake remembrances dance over our skin and leave their frigid design imprinted on our open, wounded hearts.

As Christians, when we lose the ones we cherish or hear they have an illness, it cuts deep, slicing our emotions and causing a rip down the seam of our soul. But when we turn our shredded hearts back to our Redeeming Love, the One in whom our soul trusts, we find mercy, grace, and Truth—bringing us warmth from the cold and devastating tribulation. He is the One who dwells in inapproachable light and shelters us from life's inclement weather in the hope of His Son. He is the One who thaws the snow—the only Hope who melts the icicle fingers of death, disease, suffering, and loss. I find comfort and renewed trust through the words of the apostle Peter:

Beloved, do not be surprised at the fiery ordeal among you, which comes upon you for your testing, as though some strange thing were happening to you; but to the degree that you share the sufferings of Christ, keep on rejoicing, so that also at the revelation of His glory you may rejoice with exultation.

– 1 Peter 4:12-13

He is the only One who provides the blanket as we come in from the blizzard of comatose grief. He is the Flame and Heat that soothes our chilled hearts, our Tower of Imminent Strength.

The name of the Lord is a strong tower; The righteous runs into it and is safe.

–Proverbs 18:10

He melts us with His majestic love; His Word instills us with faith and true healing that help us awaken instead of hibernating with saddened souls. As our providential provision, God gives us the courage to come out of our cave, so we can finally see and feel the springtime of living again. So, let the Light of the World be your haven when the trials of the bitter, biting winters of testing come your way: "Christian, remember the good of God in the frost of adversity" (Charles H. Spurgeon).

THE JOY OF THE LORD

Fixing our eyes on Jesus, the author and perfecter of faith, who for the joy set before Him endured the cross, despising the shame, and has sat down at the right hand of the throne of God.

– Hebrews 12:2

"God sweetens outward pain with inward peace."
– Thomas Watson

I've watched others around me suffering with various diseases and disabilities. And I've watched their souls find contentment—comfort and joy—even within the agony and distress of the disease they're battling. Cancer, rheumatoid arthritis, multiple sclerosis, heart defects, auto immune diseases, Lyme disease, Angelman syndrome, and other diseases or disabilities are just a few that haunt the people I cherish. I see friends, brothers and sisters in Christ, who were well yet now once again find themselves in the clutches of a condition that wears them down. I've watched parents raising a special needs child, clinging to the Exalted One while they walk with their child, day in and day out, through the ravages of a physically aging genetic disorder. I have a treasured friend—a mom and pastor's wife—who serves faithfully while continuously living the example of a Proverbs 31 woman. Without grumbling, she sees others as more important than herself, even though she carries multiple sclerosis in her body. I've watched a sister in Christ pray and remain at peace as her ten-year-old niece endures countless treatments of radiation and its agonizing effects; and even though the treatment assaults the young child's body—and the cancer persists—my friend continues to pray and trust God for the girl's salvation. I've watched a special friend who is a pediatric nurse fall in love with a newborn patient who, left unnurtured and abandoned at the hospital due to his fatal heart defect, became her son through the gift of adoption. Each day she trusted God for his life and trained him in the ways of the Lord, knowing he had a terminal beating heart, until the day God took him home.

While suffering as believers in Jesus Christ, so many friends surrounding me are continuing to count it all joy while the Lord keeps His hand upon them, pressing them deeper and holding them up to the fire as He refines them. No matter your situation, just like so many in my life, you can rejoice at the one thing we all have in common: *". . . the joy of the Lord is your strength"* (Nehemiah 8:10).

Paul encourages us: *"For I consider that the sufferings of this present time are not worthy to be compared with the glory that is to be revealed to us"* (Romans 8:18).

BE LIKE ZACCHEUS

Sweet friend, I wrote this book for you and for me. If you have a disease or disability, or if you are the caregiver of one who does, then you know the unceasing pain that seeks to control your life, heart, emotions, attitude, and mind. I hope and pray you keeping reading here, soaking in the encouragement like a wet sponge. I wrote this book as someone who is not a spectator of illness but a participant in a protracted, always-present disease. I live with chronic, ongoing symptoms; I grapple and wrestle with acute pain daily, yet never without hope, never without rejoicing in the Lord, and never without the deep trust and expectation of one day being part of the kingdom not of this world. When you read this book, no matter what you're facing health-wise, trial-wise, long or short, I pray you know the saving faith of Jesus Christ. I pray that your mind and heart will be renewed to see your suffering in view of God's purposes, and that you will live in gleeful anticipation, on your tiptoes like Zaccheus, who finally climbed a tree just for a glimpse of Christ:

He entered Jericho and was passing through. And there was a man
called by the name of Zaccheus; he was a chief tax collector and he
was rich. Zaccheus was trying to see who Jesus was, and was unable
because of the crowd, for he was small in stature. So he ran on ahead
and climbed up into a sycamore tree in order to see Him, for He was
about to pass through that way. When Jesus came to the place, He
looked up and said to him, "Zaccheus, hurry and come down, for
today I must stay at your house." And he hurried and came down
and received Him gladly.

– Luke 19:1-6

We can be ecstatic in the promise that Christ will one day perfect
our bodies when we meet Him in glory. This trial, this chosen path,
will lead into His everlasting kingdom.

THE RESCUER

It's hard to think of another word for "disease." It is what it is.
Describing it brings no relief in understanding its purpose from a
worldly perspective. No justice prevails in the uncouth ways it moves
about in people's bodies; and what you see isn't always what you get.
Our outer appearance can fool others into thinking we must be "fine,"
as we hear comments like, "You look good today!" For some of us, the
way we look on the outside is the exact opposite of what's going on
inside our tangled make up. No one can see inside your body to glimpse
the disease or disability trying to hold you hostage. But, friend, you
have a Defender, a Rescuer of your infirmity: Jesus Christ.

With or without disease, your body is fearfully and wonderfully
made, as David exhorts us:

I will give thanks to You, for I am fearfully and wonderfully made;
Wonderful are Your works, And my soul knows it very well.
– Psalm 139:14

And, Christ will guide you on His path if you have placed your faith and trust in Him.

Trust in the Lord with all your heart And do not lean on your
own understanding. In all your ways acknowledge Him, And He
will make your paths straight.
– Proverbs 3:5-6

Disease can make you feel as though you'll never be free. We yearn in aching urgency for it to be gone, vanished. We yearn for the torment and suffering to be no more. We long to breathe a sigh of relief, knowing we're no longer sick but healed and cured, finally experiencing the solitude of sought-after freedom and tranquil rest.

We want to live a normal life, but this is not the way for us. Our lives are far from how a typical Christian woman experiences her days. We see women who are healthy moms and wives always moving at their desired speed, flitting from one agenda to another: making grocery trips, running errands, cheering on kiddos at weekend ball games, working at jobs, rising on Sunday morning and getting the family ready for church, sometimes not thinking twice about others living in the shadow of sickness and ever-present disease or disability. We see healthy women transition from normal daytime tasks to another regiment of nightly routines: preparing dinner and doing the dishes, helping kids with homework, tucking kids in with bedtime prayers, going for a nighttime jog, and then falling soundly asleep, awakened by the alarm clock's voice to begin the next normal day. We imagine them as busy "Christian June Cleavers" while desiring their disease-free life and responsibilities.

For you it's different. Every day when you wake up, I know what you face. I know what it's like. I understand that you wear the heavy-laden coat of stringent physical and/or emotional agony and what feels like the fleece of deplorable suffering. Disease envelops and wraps itself around us like a thick, woolen layer. We cannot shed its covering when the sun shines; the binding remains. The top button chokes our neck, stifling and consuming. Our unyielding, binding overlay holds our body captive to what feels like a frozen season of life. I know what it's like to have a plaguing, hurtful, and ailing malady—a disease that makes me want to throw off its coat and dance, and yes, to just keep dancing.

We're on a Chronic Journey, and some days we will walk, some days we will skip, some days we will trip and fall, but hopefully, every day, we will have our moments to dance. Sisters, if you have a disease or disability, then you know your body doesn't always or maybe has never offered you the physical ability to twirl outside in a frilly party dress. We are not able to kick up our heels and run across the open fields like Julie Andrews in the beloved *Sound of Music*. Physically, we may be unable, but spiritually, we are alive in Christ, and we died to sin through God's gift of salvation!

Even so consider yourselves to be dead to sin, but alive to God in
Christ Jesus.
– Romans 6:11

We can have that praise and joy that dances in our souls. Every day we should choose joy and choose to let our souls dance because He has set us free from sin:

*Knowing this, that our old self was crucified with Him, in order that
our body of sin might be done away with, so that we would no longer
be slaves to sin; for he who has died is freed from sin.*
– Romans 6:6-7

Friends, we should want to dance every day in the summertime
of this life. We should long to sway back and forth, spinning around
carefree with arms out and ears piqued, taking in the rhapsody of
God's glorious creation, the background chorale of nature's crooning.
Can you imagine the wind brushing against our hale, happy cheeks,
squishing the silky grass between bare toes, knowing that feeling of
finally being free, truly free, and seeing life no more in the physical
realm? We would no longer think on the physical plight of our abiding
disease or disability but instead think on the eternal, what is to come
and what will be. These are a few of my favorite words:

*Then I saw a new heaven and a new earth; for the first heaven and
the first earth passed away, and there is no longer any sea. And
I saw the holy city, new Jerusalem, coming down out of heaven
from God, made ready as a bride adorned for her husband. And I
heard a loud voice from the throne, saying, "Behold, the tabernacle
of God is among men, and He will dwell among them, and they
shall be His people, and God Himself will be among them, and He
will wipe away every tear from their eyes; and there will no longer
be any death; there will no longer be any mourning, or crying, or
pain; the first things have passed away."
And He who sits on the throne said, "Behold, I am making all things
new." And He said, "Write, for these words are faithful and true.*
– Revelation 21:1-5

Our spiritual life in Him is the source of your freedom. Do not let
your physical life and disability or disease dictate how you live your

spiritual life. Don't hide in the bleachers at the high school dance. Dance with me. Dance for Christ in your heart. Come along with me, and dance. Step out with your whole soul. Today and for the rest of your life, let your soul dance and your heart be filled with praise for the Creator—a heart that looks like that of our Lord.

A PROCLAMATION

This book is a proclamation of God's resounding and biblical affection to those who suffer every moment of every day with a sustained disease, condition, or disability—one that oftentimes tries to erode your heart and keep you in the yawning pass, stuck and no longer willing or trying to make it through, simply stagnant. The God of Mercy has a limitless love for all those He adopts and ushers in as His tender kin; He is your Father if you've been adopted and grafted into His family:

> *Blessed be the God and Father of our Lord Jesus Christ, who has blessed us with every spiritual blessing in the heavenly places in Christ, just as He chose us in Him before the foundation of the world, that we would be holy and blameless before Him. In love He predestined us to adoption as sons through Jesus Christ to Himself, according to the kind intention of His will, to the praise of the glory of His grace, which he freely bestowed on us in the Beloved.*
> – Ephesians 1:3-6

He is the One who heals, comforts, and repairs and who gives us the binding spiritual contract that never dies. He is the stout and firm Ancestral Tree. He is our strong, faithful Vine, and we are His branches.

*I am the vine, you are the branches; he who abides in Me and I in
him, he bears much fruit, for apart from Me you can do nothing.*
– John 15:5

He is the One who hung on that purposed wood. He is the One
who gives us a never-failing compassion as a Faithful Ruler who commands us to run. He tells us to run as to win the prize.
*Do you not know that those who run in a race all run, but only one
receives the prize? Run in such a way that you may win.*
– 1 Corinthians 9:24

So, run with worth unmerited, strive without angst, because you
have placed the yoke on Him.
*Take My yoke upon you and learn from Me, for I am gentle and
humble in heart, and YOU WILL FIND REST FOR YOUR SOULS.*
– Matthew 11:29

Once a newborn on milk, you should now be growing up in your
faith and living on the meat of His Word.
*Like newborn babies, long for the pure milk of the word, so that by it
you may grow in respect to salvation, if you have tasted the kindness
of the Lord.*
–1 Peter 2:2-3

His Word gives us spiritual eyes to see the finish line, the golden
streets that await us, if you are His beloved. Jehovah-Jireh means "The
Lord Will Provide," and He does, truly, lavish us with an incomprehensible, unseen, beneficial love. His affection is forgiving, never keeping
record of all the corruptness and sin we've committed. He willingly
lowered Himself into the dark earth and felt the stark, temporal hold

of death, but because He is the I AM, it could not contain Him, and He rose miraculously so He could keep His boundless assertion. Christ's agape-bond is relentless—pursuing us and then transforming us.

But we all, with unveiled face, beholding as in a mirror the glory of the Lord, are being transformed into the same image from glory to glory, just as from the Lord, the Spirit.

– 2 Corinthians 3:18

As believing sisters, we are united to Him in death but risen with Him in new life, salvific life. It is superhuman, a worthy allegiance that cannot be thwarted, but is forever, as one day when the sky is rolled up like a scroll, we will stand before Him, praising Him forevermore, without disease and disability. Our putrid, earthly bodies will then be cloaked in royal garments, pure and healed, performing a new chorus of worship, singing anthems of "all things made new." That melodic soul will be you, and so with each breath, fill your lungs and use them to worship, singing songs of praise and hymns of hope, telling of His wonders and mercy.

Shout joyfully to the Lord, all the earth; Break forth and sing for joy and sing praises.

– Psalm 98:4

This is your book as well as mine. It's the account of strong, amazing women who bear disease or disability and who can rejoice through this temporal and, at times, suffering-filled life by understanding the love of Christ. The only way to love Christ is to know Christ and be known by Him.

And we know that the Son of God has come, and has given us under-standing so that we may know Him who is true; and we are in Him who is true, in His Son Jesus Christ. This is the true God and eternal life.

– 1 John 5:20

I am the good shepherd, and I know My own and My own know Me.
— John 10:14

We know Christ by repenting of our sin and making Him our Lord and Savior. We grow in the faith of the saints by sitting at the foot of the Teacher with a soul crying out to be pristine—shined and buffed in the light of His Word. By reading the Bible, studying it, and applying it to our lives, His Holy Book becomes our truth compass, pointing us home to the foot of the cross. By following Christ, we live at the foot of the soul-mending, joy-unending, life-giving cross.

THE LETTER

Disease can manifest as a personal, heavy, and corroding insignia for each of us. For me, it was a bittersweet, tough-love letter stamped, sealed, and mailed to me at the age of twenty-two. The correspondence sent to my soul, written before the foundation of the world, declared that God had chosen me for a trial that would test my faith in a way I could have never foreseen; the letter was written in words I understood, prompting me to want to return it to my faithful Sender. But it was mine to keep, and that's when the real journey began—the journey of transformation, of looking a bit more like Christ, taxing and tearing me, teaching me about a God who would instruct me by His Word.

I will meditate on Your precepts And regard Your ways. I shall delight in Your statutes; I shall not forget Your Word.
— Psalm 119:15-16

As I read this letter with tear-stained eyes, I saw that my greatest freedom rested in being His follower, His beloved child—I was finally free! I was freed from my captivity, from my bondage of sin and no longer at the hands of a merciless disease, by being a slave to Christ. My footprints were left on the weathered but straight and narrow path that I walked, and finding His strength moment by moment, not veering to the right or left. I learned to pick up my pace and continue to walk by faith daily.

For we walk by faith, not by sight.

– 2 Corinthians 5:7

By reading each page of God's Word, I discovered more and more about my journey and the plan my God designed, the road He paved, the path He carved out. A drawn out, significant walk He has chosen for me—one that proves humbly engaging, loud yet tranquil, comfortable yet cumbersome, mysterious yet poignant, and tiresome yet satisfying—and I continue on it daily.

THE LEADING PATH

The Lord's path for my life stretches out distinct, and His path for you does as well. In all this earth, first and foremost, we are to bring Him glory.

Not to us, O Lord, not to us,
But to Your name give glory Because of Your lovingkindness, because
of Your truth.

– Psalm 115:1

No one else has the same road marked out the exact same way. All of us have different triumphs, miseries, joys, and trials; our providential lifespan is unique to each of us. If you're a child of the Most High, of the God who cares for the brokenhearted, of the One who bore the shame of our stain-infested souls, then this path you're on was tailor-made before the foundation of the world, specifically for and only for you. It's crafted unique to strip away your old "man"—the unredeemed man or vagabond who carried his knapsack on the dusty, dirty road leading to Hell. And it's custom-designed to keep you ever-closer to Him.

A GOOD PLAN

God's plan is for your spiritual good, as the apostle Paul so fervently reminds us.

And we know that God causes all things to work together for good to those who love God, to those who are called according to His purpose.
– Romans 8:28

The "good" Paul describes here is spiritual; God advances the good plan for our lives as we are given salvation and become more like Him. Your life in Christ is marked by spiritual growth—maturing in Truth and knowledge as a new woman, no longer tattered and unclean, but now refreshed and new. In this verse, our Messiah is talking about the good we've been given as we are given salvation. You can't touch it or see it because it's spiritual. The great good of salvation is your redemption through the Gospel. "Good" doesn't mean that everything happening to you illustrates a motivational quote posted on a Facebook page. That's fantasy. Physically, we won't always come out smelling like roses. We must endure persecution, pain, struggle with sin, injustice, betrayal, death, and loss. With a disease or disability, we sometimes walk through what feels like an infinity of suffering and, at times, unlimited torment, both physical and emotional. You're learning to live with disease just as I am, trusting and knowing that God purposed it.

The LORD will accomplish what concerns me; Your lovingkindness,
O Lord, is everlasting; Do not forsake the works of Your hands.
     – Psalm 138:8

You've probably encountered many thorny trials because of the enduring hinderance of disease or disability, but these trials are making you bloom, serving as a crowning floret. Growth comes with thorns and necessitates you stand in the scorching sun, fraught with drought, and then endure a downpour of pounding rain, creating a soil in which no other flower could survive. These elements make us fight for life and fight for a stem that can stand. We need petals that hold up when the rains keep coming—as flowers that radiate beauty in a tended garden, as blooms that survive and thrive by the tender hand of the master Gardner. Our God is the One who tills the soil and causes us to grow up in the newness of spiritual birth.

Blessed be the God and Father of our Lord Jesus Christ, who according to His great mercy has caused us to be born again to a living hope through the resurrection of Jesus Christ from the dead.
     – 1 Peter 1:3

GOD'S GIFTS

When you were a child, Christmas was all about gifts. Many children know that once the tree is up, it's present time. Presents start appearing one by one. On Christmas Day, when they finally tear into each package, kids discover that some of the gifts are ones included on their list and some are "parent picks." In children's minds, toys beat socks and clothes any day, but those items are needed. Some gifts are too big, and kids must grow into them. Some gifts don't suit their style or taste, and they may dread wearing them in public; but parents give presents for their children's good. Kids may not want them, but parents know what's best. And it's the same with God's gifts. They're always good, full of His love and sweet care, but sometimes not wrapped up in pretty pink packages tied up with string; they're not what we want or expect.

I never expected disease. I never expected to see my disease as a gift, but these kinds of purposed trials and loving "parent picks" are what make us more like Christ.

> *And if children, heirs also, heirs of God and fellow heirs with*
> *Christ, if indeed we suffer with Him so we may also be glorified*
> *with Him. For I consider that the sufferings of this present time are*
> *not worthy to be compared with the glory that is to be revealed to us.*
> – Romans 8:17-18

Because of God's ultimate plan, we know that if we're in Christ, His gracious favor and lush, steadfast love cling to our soul like the dewy honey on the wafers of a bee's comb. And, He is with us as we walk through life with this sticky bout!

> *You, O Lord, will not withhold Your compassion from me;*
> *Your lovingkindness and Your truth will continually preserve me.*
> *For evils beyond number have surrounded me;*
> *My iniquities have overtaken me, so that I am not able to see;*
> *They are more numerous than the hairs of my head,*
> *And my heart has failed me*
> *Be pleased, O Lord, to deliver me.*
> *Make haste, O Lord, to help me.*
> – Psalm 40:11-13

I SURRENDER ALL ... OH, TO THEE, MY BLESSED SAVIOR, I SURRENDER ALL

Some of you are ready to surrender all the weighted yoke of disease or disability that wants to impede your walk, your worship, and your shackled soul from wanting to praise Him. For some of us, the yoke is unbearable. We have so much sin baggage, but Christ tells us to repent and that He will make our yoke light.

For My yoke is easy and My burden is light.

– Matthew 11:30

Some of us need encouragement, rebuke, and correction to help us repent of our cut-throat anger, longstanding bitterness, and lowest mortification of anguish that has painted our grief so black. And some of us just need lots of soul hugs and kisses to be reminded we are alive in Christ—and must leave our worries and sin luggage at the claims desk and board the right flight, sit down in first class, and live in obedience to Christ.

THE DEEP VALLEY

As you are hiking on this steep and rocky ravine, trekking on an unclear quest and facing earthly erosion, you're being sanctified. *"Then THE RIGHTEOUS WILL SHINE FORTH AS THE SUN in the kingdom of their Father. He who has ears, let him hear"* (Matthew 13:43).

I know how disease tries to dissolve your spirit and flesh without reprieve. I know the feeling of your emotions rubbing raw, the pain suffocating, and the ravine more treacherous today than before; your eyes feel hazy as you strain to see the thin trail—but keep taking steps. Stay on the path! You're still breathing, and as you open your eyes each morning, continue to spiritually put one foot in front of the other, using your voice to worship Him because He is the God of the deep ravine as well as the lush plains.

Will you praise Him on the crown pinnacle of the mountain but not in the deeps of the fathomless valley? Will you praise Him in the times of despair as well as exuberance, with disease or without, when you're empty as well as giddy? Will you lift up your praise when you feel like it and when you don't, with or without your earnest prayers and desires fulfilled, in all seasons of life, when He gives and when He takes away? *"The Lord gave and the Lord has taken away. Blessed be the name of the Lord"* (Job 1:21b).

In all our circumstances with disease, even as gut wrenching as the toll it places on our body and mind, He demands our acclaim and whole-hearted worship. Morning and evening praise the Lord. As the psalmist states, I consider it a privilege *"To declare Your lovingkindness in the morning and Your faithfulness by night"* (Psalm 92:2). Walking, jumping, crawling, trudging, or climbing out of the seemingly impossible ravines, you will make it. You will always make it—in the ravine, in the trials—if you're a follower of Christ and your faith is the rock on which you're standing.

> *One thing I have asked from the Lord, that I shall seek:*
> *That I may dwell in the house of the Lord all the days of my life,*
> *To behold the beauty of the Lord*
> *And to meditate in His temple.*
> *For in the day of trouble He will conceal me in His tabernacle;*
> *In the secret place of His tent He will hide me;*
> *He will lift me up on a rock.*
> *– Psalm 27:4-5*

So, stick your flag in the ground and stake your claim: your claim on trusting; your claim to walk through the parted Red Sea and the valley of the shadow of death; your claim to not look back like Lot's wife did, with fear and what ifs; your claim to put the Lord before all else, to put your Heavenly Father before your family, friends, your desires, and even your disease. Now is the time to live for the cross. Now is the time to stake your claim and live for Him.

> *For am I now seeking the favor of men, or of God? Or am I striving*
> *to please men? If I were still trying to please men, I would not be*
> *a bond-servant of Christ.*
>
> – Galatians 1:10

Knowing that God loves you with that kind of a profound love should draw your misted eyes upward. We should be overcome, amazed by a called Love, a divine gift of life that tore the veil. *"And behold, the veil of the temple was torn in two from top to bottom; and the earth shook and the rocks were split"* (Matthew 27:51).

His sacrificial love should cause our souls to overflow with praise and us to bow in humble adoration. There is no other love that would or could do what Christ did on the cross: He gave His own life, so you and I would have eternal life. Christ is our abiding Love.

A MUG OF CHERISHED JAVA

I wrote this book candidly as if you were sitting here with me, sipping a hot cup of coffee, soaking in a long-anticipated morning, as the sun peeks up its head. This is a visit with two best friends, two kindred spirits who need to catch up and can speak God's Truth into each other's life. We are sisters who can relate, cry together, pray together, and study the Bible together.

> *Blessed be the God and Father of our Lord Jesus Christ, the Father of*
> *mercies and God of all comfort, who comforts us in all our affliction*
> *so that we will be able to comfort those who are in any affliction*
> *with the comfort with which we ourselves are comforted by God.*
>
> – 2 Corinthians 1:3-4

Just like coffee often tastes better with sugar and cream well stirred, so do genuine friends make us alive like pepped up joe. With loyal friends, we're not just a cup of plain black coffee but a warm mug of cherished java. So, I ask you, my cup of java and gracious friend, find a cozy spot, nestle in, and let's talk heart to heart as we begin our time together on this life venture. I pray that you see your life story, or that of someone you care for or know, here in these pages, and I hope in my heart that you believe in the comfort of a never-ending, saving love that only God bestows: His salvation in Jesus Christ alone.

> *And the testimony is this, that God has given us eternal life, and this life is in His Son. He who has the Son has the life; he who does not have the Son of God does not have the life. These things I have written to you who believe in the name of the Son of God, so that you may know that you have eternal life.*
>
> – 1 John 5:11-13

LEARNING AND LIVING AS A CHRONIC CHRISTIAN

Throughout this book, my sister, we will focus on what it means to live with a brutal disease and how we find our counsel, encouragement, and instruction in our Sovereign God's Word. We will focus on these things to teach us to live in joy and anticipation of our Redeemer's return, suffer righteously, flee temptation, and find comfort and hope in Scripture. It will show us our sin and point us back to the Keeper of Our Soul. As sisters in Christ, He will give us hope to endure our physical pain. We will learn to continuously keep our eyes on the prize of the next life. *"I press on toward the goal for the prize of the upward call of God in Christ Jesus"* (Philippians 3:14).

I pray it will give you, as well as your caregiver, strength and comfort; you are not alone. Our own God suffered and felt punishing travail and torture and was crucified on Calvary's cross. He is our awesome help amid the mad river of life, the One to whom every knee will bow, the One who gives everlasting life to those who belong to Him. He is the One who showers His children with the closest affection of all: a forever, loyal, fixed-in-place love and everlasting peace in Heaven with perfect bodies.

I pray if you're a believer that this will encourage, strengthen, challenge, and grow you in your daily walk with our Creator—and if you've arrived at this page without knowing the Savior, that you will come to know Him. I realize that some of you may have just had a child or loved one recently diagnosed with a disease, or maybe you're the one just diagnosed; maybe you've been struggling for years with disease or disability or you know someone who has. Friend, my heart is joined with yours, and I kneel on my knees offering up supplication for you. Even though I don't know you, I hope you will consider me a forever friend, a cherished mug of java. I am a sister in Christ who can understand, a devout companion who suffers with you. God does not change.

> *God is not a man, that He should lie, Nor a son of man, that He should repent; Has He said, and will He not do it? Or has He spoken, and will He not make it good?*
> – Numbers 23:19

He is immutable. He will always give you the strength you need; His Word will always provide the counsel and wisdom you need through these trials. *"But if any of you lacks wisdom, let him ask of God, who gives to all generously and without reproach, and it will be given to him"* (James 1:5).

He will always be with us and never stop loving us, even in our disease or disability. He is the Alpha and Omega, the same from the beginning to endless eternity.

Scripture tells us to hope in the promise that, one day, all the pain and suffering will be no more. One day, we will reign with him in eternity, released from this fallen world, this broken body, this gritty struggle. Sisters, in this book you will find there is Hope and eternal life in Jesus Christ and Him alone. As a Christian woman, I pray this book gives you a depth of His amazing grace, a new, vigorous endurance through the Truth, and a desire to face your disease or disability with the boldness of a well decorated soldier. So, lift your eyes to the mountains; He is where we find our Help:

> *I will lift up my eyes to the mountains;*
> *From where shall my help come?*
> *My help comes from the Lord,*
> *Who made heaven and earth.*
> *He will not allow your foot to slip;*
> *He who keeps you will not slumber.*
> *Behold, He who keeps Israel*
> *Will neither slumber nor sleep.*
> – Psalm 121:1-4

If you do not know the salvation found only in Christ, I pray that through this book and hearing the Gospel, you receive new life: Life in Christ. He is the only One who can love you with a Chronic Love! By book's end, may you know the truth and sacrificial merit in Christ, our Lord and Savior. So, let's begin together. Praise God! Come quickly, Lord Jesus, come!

Loving Father,

I pray for all the women, young and old, who are beginning this Chronic Journey of disease and trusting You with Your plans for their lives. Lord, please also comfort those who have had to see a loved one pass from this earth and are grieving the agonizing loss. Help them to find peace and rest in your arms. I pray you would give them the strength they need to endure the pain of living without their loved one. You are our only Truth and Strength. Lord, I pray for those women long suffering with disease, who have been deep in the valley of pain or know someone who is—please give them grace and show them your goodness and give them the peace that surpasses all understanding. As we begin this Chronic Journey of learning how to live with disease or disability, help our minds through this book to be renewed and changed. Give us wisdom and teach and mold our hearts as we find our only dependence in You. As we read these chapters, may we find our only hope in You, receiving fresh eyes and faith to walk through this trial. In Jesus' holy name I pray . . .

Amen!

Chapter Two

CHRIST'S CHRONIC LOVE THROUGH SALVATION

*"Atonement by the blood of Jesus is not an arm of Christian truth;
it is the heart of it."*
– Charles Spurgeon

*I have been crucified with Christ; and it is no longer I who live, but
Christ lives in me; and the life I now live in the flesh I live by faith in
the Son of God, who loved me and gave Himself up for me.*
– Galatians 2:20

Dear Precious Sister,

In Chapter One you learned about the journey you're taking through this book and what to expect along the way. As we unfold each of the next chapters, I want you to view chronic as a word that gives hope to life, wings to the earthbound, food to the famished, a melody to the song-less, and a jeweled tiara to a reigning princess. Yes, we are the princesses of the world, the fair maidens of the fairytale that ends Happily Ever After if we know the Chronic Christ. Do not view your disease or disability as filled with hopelessness and unrest; that's the old definition of chronic.

The word chronic has never received a positive connotation; it's never been considered your welcomed guest or best friend but, instead, an enemy who clings to your disease and sucks the life from your flesh, imprisoning you like a confined ball and chain. Please know this: the word chronic is not our nemesis and not our volatile enemy; not today, not in this book, and not ever again. It no longer exists as the integral link to the name and kind of disease or disability you find yourself battling.

You no longer embody the face you see in the mirror: the sometimes face of sadness, confusion, and exhaustion that peers back at you from framed glass hanging on your wall. No more! From now on, impress the word chronic on your heart and ingrain it in your mind as a word associated with hope, salvation, faith, and the Word of God. The meaning of this word is no longer burdened by shame of negative proportions but signifies a lasting freedom. It's a word that points to the hope, salvation, and peace found only in Christ. See it as an antique mirror, like one chiseled with roses around its edges that sits on your vanity—the mirror that you can't wait to look into each morning. See yourself in this mirror as one beheld anew, invigorated and full of goodness through His Word and Spirit.

Now . . . if your body allows you to do so . . . put on your makeup, brush back your hair, and let's restart the day. And if your body doesn't allow you to accomplish the daily, physical acts of life, remember that we as believers can still look in the mirror of our heart and spiritually live and breathe for Him. We can daily groom our hearts for the consecrated bridegroom:

> *I will rejoice greatly in the* Lord,
> *My soul will exult in my God;*
> *For He has clothed me with garments of salvation,*
> *He has wrapped me with a robe of righteousness,*

As a bridegroom decks himself with a garland,
And as a bride adorns herself with her jewels.
– Isaiah 61:10

SALVATION

I know you suffer, I know you hurt, but a way is available for you to live this life with joy. There is a way to live this life with contentment. It's not a pill, magic potion, or quote by Oprah hanging on the fridge; it's not karma, or yoga, or meditation. My precious friend, your contentment is not found in fad diets, essential oils, a Christian women's conference, or a higher calling or purpose; and it does not lie in money, exotic vacations, or a "name it and claim it" healing. The secret to living this life is "through Christ," the God-man who came down to us, who lived here on earth to give His life as a ransom for many.

"For even the Son of Man did not come to be served, but to serve, and
to give His life as a ransom for many."
– Mark 10:45

As my pastor says, "God treated Christ as if He had lived my sinful, guilty life so that He could treat me as if I had lived Christ's perfect life."

As you begin this chapter, understand that my constant desire is steeped in your everlasting, forever-eternal salvation. My prayer is for you to become a true follower of our Lord and Savior, Jesus Christ, the immutable, immortal God. He is the One who saves us from our sin.

"In this is love, not that we loved God, but that He loved us and sent
His Son to be the propitiation for our sins."
– 1 John 4:10

Jesus Christ remains the God of the universe, the true and living God. He is the only One who can help you perfectly through this trial and the persistent physical and mental pain of bearing a chronic disease or disability. Without believing in Christ for salvation, you will be lost in this crass culture. It means you will agree with the world's system and beliefs and find yourself fighting in your own power as you walk around like a compliant robot limited to rigid motions. Without Christ, your disease or disability and the sin inside you dictate who you are and let you sink away in the quicksand of worldly views and false hope, a dead life. A life lived without Christ is life without joy inexpressible, without the gracious and granted faith with which He supplies us; a life without Christ is one devoid of a faith that can take a giant like Goliath and knock him to the ground with nothing but a slingshot, a pebble, and a tiny boy with a heart after God.

> Then David said to the Philistine, "You come to me with a sword, a spear, and a javelin, but I come to you in the name of the Lord of hosts, the God of the armies of Israel, whom you have taunted. This day the Lord will deliver you up into my hands . . ." Then it happened when the Philistine rose and came and drew near to meet David, that David ran quickly toward the battle line to meet the Philistine. And David put his hand into his bag and took from it a stone and slung it and struck the Philistine on his forehead. And the stone sank into his forehead, so that he fell on his face to the ground . . . When the Philistines saw that their champion was dead, they fled.
>
> – 1 Samuel 17:45-46, 48-49, 51

Salvation is the truth and it's free, as free as a bird taking flight. Without life in Christ, you will someday come to the end of the time He's given you and, having rejected Him, you will then spend eternity forever in Hell, wracked with gnashing pain.

"In that place there will be weeping and gnashing of teeth when you see Abraham and Isaac and Jacob and all the prophets in the king-dom of God, but yourselves being thrown out."

– Luke 13:28

Without life in Christ, you will be severed from the inimitable, immortal, majestic Messiah.

THE REAL DEAL: THE REAL LIFE

In this chapter, we will talk about the meaning and gift of salvation. Salvation has been given to you by Christ so that you will know—with-out a doubt—that your life has hope, that you have a Protector . . . a Friend . . . a Father . . . a Savior who loves you. Your life with Christ is no longer void of light but full of the Light who came into this dark world.

"He who sees Me sees the One who sent Me. I have come as Light into the world, so that everyone who believes in Me will not remain in darkness."

– John 12:45-46

He is the Light of Salvation, a Love that acquits a bound-up soul, a Love that gives unending life, not just for 1,000 or 5,000, or 10,000 years, but for *eternity*! God used Christ the Son as the saint-key to turn the lock in the cell block door, flinging open the gates of heaven instead of keeping you forged behind the clanking bars of an eternal jail cell. When you receive His gift of Life, freeing you from sin, He gives you the real deal: the real life!

Before we go any further, let's look at our journey through this book by solidifying your understanding of the Gospel's meaning and significance. Without the Gospel, we are without hope, dead before we're even placed in a casket, with a man-centered eulogy and a blank tombstone. Why do we choose to be defunct, spiritless zombies? Why do we want to encapsulate the walking dead in this life, facing disease without the Bread of Life feeding our souls and making us alive in the here and now? In this life before salvation, we are stumbling around mindless and looking for everything but Christ to satisfy our fleshly carnage. We are a worldly, temporal carcass of dry and dead bones. Why would we want to be effectually dead when we can be given viable lifeblood from the Love-Sacrifice Himself?

". . . and not through the blood of goats and calves, but through
His own blood, He entered the holy place once for all, having ob-
tained eternal redemption."

– Hebrews 9:12

How do we receive the second birth? His promise to give us new birth "by the Spirit" is explained to us as Christ talks to Nicodemus, the rich, worldly member of the Jewish Sanhedrin who is willing to associate with Christ only by the canopy of night, until he becomes a faithful disciple and proudly identifies Jesus as the Light. These words of John explain this truth:

This is the message we have heard from Him and announce to you,
that God is Light, and in Him there is no darkness at all. If we say
that we have fellowship with Him and yet walk in the darkness,
we lie and do not practice the truth; but if we walk in the Light as He
Himself is in the Light, we have fellowship with one another, and the

blood of Jesus His Son cleanses us from all sin. If we say that we have
no sin, we are deceiving ourselves and the truth is not in us.
                                        – 1 John 1:5-8

Before Nicodemus makes such a drastic transformation as a true follower, he is looking for the answer to how a grown man is born a second time. How can a man be born when he is old?

> Nicodemus said to Him, "How can a man be born when he is old? He cannot enter a second time into his mother's womb and be born, can he?" Jesus answered, "Truly, truly, I say to you, unless one is born of water and the Spirit he cannot enter into the kingdom of God. That which is born of the flesh is flesh, and that which is born of the Spirit is spirit. Do not be amazed that I said to you, 'You must be born again.' The wind blows where it wishes and you hear the sound of it, but do not know where it comes from and where it is going; so is everyone who is born of the Spirit."
>
> – John 3:4-8

Christ tells him how to become a spiritual infant. How can we be born again into a living and breathing heart and soul? The answer is the same for Nicodemus those thousands of years ago as it is for us today. Nothing has changed; being "reborn" means being regenerated by God and born of the Spirit and believing in Jesus Christ for your salvation.

So, what is the Gospel? . . . So, what is salvation? We are going to pull back the curtain of life and examine what the Bible teaches us about God's remedy for sin. We are going to learn about or be humbled again by the sacred, true love story God wrote for us—a story so powerful and so magnificent it was quilled in the crimson blood of Jesus Christ. Each page, each book and chapter of His Word, is filled with abiding atonement. The providential "Narrator and Author of Time and the Bible" loves us with an unending love, a pure love—not a fluffy, Hallmark, mushy love—but a selfless love. Our loving Father sent Christ, the Incarnate who was tortured and crucified:

> They stripped Him and put a scarlet robe on Him. And after twisting together a crown of thorns, they put it on His head, and a reed in His right hand; and they knelt down before Him and mocked Him, saying, "Hail, King of the Jews!" They spat on Him, and took the reed and began to beat Him on the head. After they had mocked Him, they took the scarlet robe off Him and put His own garments back on Him, and led Him away to crucify Him.
> – Matthew 27:28-31

As believers, He sent Christ for you and for me. We are the ones who threw stones, cursed Him, plucked down the thorny crown on His red-soaked scalp, and watched the blood surge from atop His furrowed brow. We handed the soldiers the spear to drive into His flesh-exposed side. We looked up at His lamentable face as His neck hung sunken and low, and we pointed, laughed, cursed, and waited in evil excitement for His rapid breath to cease. We stood at the cross, not for mercy, but for vengeful satisfaction. What a disheartening and utterly despicable reality that you and I were that person! You and I crucified Christ! Try to let your heart meditate on that realization. We may not have been physically there on the day the earth went pitch black and shook, when the dead wakened and walked out of their tombs, the day Christ sacrificed His life for you and me, but this alone should be enough: He laid down His life and offered up His spirit for you.

"And Jesus cried out again with a loud voice, and yielded up His spirit."
– Matthew 27:50

We could end the book right there. This is the faith to which we hold. What a grand display of unconditional love He displayed on the cross! What an astounding truth that should cause us to pick up our cross daily and die to ourselves.

"And He was saying to them all, 'If anyone wishes to come after Me, he must deny himself, and take up his cross daily and follow Me'."
– Luke 9:23

And, it's enough for us to be content with our own thorn jabbing into our flesh, the disease or disability that we live with. God's grace is sufficient for us, just as it was for Paul.

Concerning this I implored the Lord three times that it might leave me. And He has said to me, "My grace is sufficient for you, for power is perfected in weakness." Most gladly, therefore, I will rather boast about my weaknesses, so that the power of Christ may dwell in me. Therefore, I am well content with weaknesses, with insults, with distresses, with persecutions, with difficulties, for Christ's sake; for when I am weak, then I am strong."
– 2 Corinthians 12:8-10

Because of the great sacrifice Christ paid at Calvary, we are innocent, no longer a guilty or wanted criminal, but baptized into New Life through His death and resurrection.

*"Blessed be the God and Father of our Lord Jesus Christ, who accord-
ing to His great mercy has caused us to be born again to a living
hope through the resurrection of Jesus Christ from the dead . . . "*
– 1 Peter 1:3

This is the truth we cling to as Christians. As saved women who
battle disease or disability each day, we should relish the truth of the
Gospel. By reading and applying it, we have the power in His strength
to fight this disease and not let it master us.

THERE IS A FOUNTAIN

He gave those life who would come and drink from the fountain
of His blood—those who would lay down their scarlet-cloaked
rags as they waded out of the water, baptized and walking in the
purity of a cleansed soul with new garments. Do you still walk in
dingy, sin-stained clothes, or are you dressed in showy, untouched,
pure regalia? Christ is the Living Water, the perpetual life-giving
Fountain, and His untainted, living spring can clean every stain. He's
the only Fountain that can take us, each a dirty sinner, and make us
brand new. He's the vital flood who holds the power to take away the
guilt, shame, depression, anxiety, and emotional shockwaves—the
old you—and dunk you into the living water, washing away all the
sin from your born-again soul. All those empty feelings inside, all
those tar-coated sins, are forever carried away in the current of His
love and sacrifice for you. No one else can offer you this rushing,
gushing Fountain, who creates you a regenerated being.

When we're born again, we turn as white and bright as the
bleached spot on a black-as-soot T-shirt. We stand out. We are new;

we are different, a beyond-sparkling-white, like drab milk tones that suddenly take on a vibrant, eye-shielding, heavenly glow. We stand out because we're born-again beings. When Christ died on the cross, He died for those past, present, and future, for those who believed that He is God, that He is the Savior, the Promised One. He died for every sin we have or will commit. He died for the sins from our past, from before we're Christians; for the sins we commit in our present; and for the future sins we will commit as believers because we are fallen creatures. So, let's begin the true story of the God who was flesh and blood and lived and walked this earth: let's talk about the Gospel. Yes, let's face our disease head on—with the power of the scarlet geyser that quenches forever the thirst of a desolate, desert soul:

There is a fountain filled with blood
Drawn from Immanuel's veins
And sinners plunged beneath that flood
Lose all their guilty stains
Lose all their guilty stains
Lo And sinners plunged beneath that flood
Lose all their guilty stains.

– From "There Is a Fountain"
a hymn by William Cowper, written in 1772

THE GOOD NEWS OF A GOOD GOD

What is the Gospel?

The first thing we need to understand is that God is the Creator and He is over all. Genesis 1:1, the Bible's very first verse, says, *"In the beginning, God created the heavens and the earth."* It tells us that God is Creator of all and has existed since before the world and time began.

He has always been here; He has never not existed. If God is Creator, then you and I are His creations. We were made by Him.

When I look up in the sky and see the way the clouds hover, I remember how, as a little girl, I imagined them to be an elephant, or a man with a crooked nose, or a melting ice cream cone, but even then, as a young, skinny, impressionable kid, I knew there was a God. The sky was my backdrop to draw those cotton-like figures in my imagination, which eventually glided along and took on other shapes. When I look at my daughter and peer into the intricacy of her open eyes, the deep tones like the color of blanched almonds with all the richness of a glossy, satiny-smooth milk chocolate bar, I find myself asking, "Who can make those marble hues?"

Creation is everywhere. Creation is right before you; it's in the morning, waking you up, urging you to look out your window and gaze upon the way a hummingbird beats its wings so effortlessly while it awaits the sweet honey water in a feeder swinging from a branch in your backyard. When I see my newborn baby grow up each day and turn into an eight-year-old little girl who craves the morning—so she can wake up, run downstairs in her pajamas and cuddle with Mama, her hair tangled from a night of sleeping and dreaming, all smiles, with a raspy little voice and sleep dust still hiding in those big almond eyes—I see creation. The Bible tells us there is a Creator. I know God as my Marvelous Maker and so do you, even if you lie to yourself by suppressing the truth or try to excuse it away.

For since the creation of the world His invisible attributes, His eternal power and divine nature, have been clearly seen, being understood through what has been made, so that they are without excuse."
                                                              – Romans 1:20

The Bible says there is no excuse to not believe in God; He is evident through creation.

> *"He has made everything appropriate in its time. He has also set eternity in their heart, yet so that man will not find out the work which God has done from the beginning even to the end."*
>
> – Ecclesiastes 3:11

On a clear, sunny day, no one can look into the baby blue sky above and explain away the design of such an exact and precise God as our Creator:

> *O Lord, how many are Your works!*
> *In wisdom You have made them all;*
> *The earth is full of Your possessions.*
> *There is the sea, great and broad,*
> *In which are swarms without number,*
> *Animals both small and great.*
> *O Lord, how many are Your works!*
> *In wisdom You have made them all;*
> *The earth is full of Your possessions.*
> *There is the sea, great and broad,*
> *In which are swarms without number,*
> *Animals both small and great.*
>
> – Psalm 104:24-25

We see the sun by day and the chalky moon by night, and though the moon waxes and wanes and the sun sometimes shrouded in clouds, we know all happens in its appointed time; the sun rises and sets, marking the seasons, and the glowing moon offers a nightlight, like a lighthouse beacon amid a sprinkle of stars. No matter if you're a native in the aborigine jungle or a modern business woman in bustling New York, you will see the sun and the moon making their arcs across the sky—and if you take the time, you'll find yourself gaping in awe at creation's magnificence.

You can see another example of ordered creation in the way the tide rolls in. How the waves come tumbling inland reminds me of children who discover the best use for living room carpet: to practice doing a forward roll, endlessly, repeatedly. As the salty waves spiral in from the ocean to the sandy shore, day in and day out, each follows an exact, identical ordered pattern. We know the tide rises and falls at a predictable time each day, influenced by the moon and its pull on the earth. This is God's creation, His ordered timetable.

The waves were spoken into existence by our great God, and He created water to sustain our lives.

> *"Then God said, 'Let the waters below the heavens be gathered into one place, and let the dry land appear'; and it was so."*
> – Genesis 1:9

It's too much for our minds to comprehend that God created the earth in seven days, that He created life.

> *"Then God said, 'Let Us make man in Our image, according to Our likeness; and let them rule over the fish of the sea and over the birds of the sky and over the cattle and over all the earth, and over every creeping thing that creeps on the earth.'"*
> – Genesis 1:26

The earth is His creation; we are made in His image.

> *"God created man in His own image, in the image of God He created him; male and female He created them."*
> – Genesis 1:27

Not one of us can refute the miracle of conception, life given by the Life-Giver Himself, who gives the soul a reason to be born. Evidence of His handiwork shines all around us. We are His evidence. Each one of us has a one-of-a-kind talent and unique set of abilities. We possess different mixes of personality traits, we exude different emotions, and our physical appearance is created unique. No two people look exactly alike; even twins possess uniqueness all their own. All of us develop different likes and dislikes, different tastes, in our music, clothes, food choices . . . yes, even our taste buds are formed distinct. We are complex and multi-faceted, all the way down to individual nuances, such as how we sound when we laugh. Each uniquely crafted person provides evidence that we are intricately designed by a personal, loving Being—the God of the universe. The Bible makes it clear: we have no excuse to not know that the Creator is the Lord.

If our Creator did not personally take time to design each of us with variant individuality, we would all look the same and think in unison. We would all be in sync, clones marching in lockstep. But instead, we're all beautifully different, portraits of a set-apart love. Some people are tall; some short. Different skin tones, races, and nationalities—even different bodies—grace the world. Some people are physically in shape and hit the gym daily, and some are incurably sick. Some can walk while some are disabled. Infants are being welcomed into their mom's cradling posture; bodybuilders with strong, chiseled muscles are bench pressing colossal weights; and others are walking feebly, canes in hand to cross the hospital doorway for their next radiation treatment. There are women who seem to hold the key to the fountain of youth in their genes, while others age rapidly, their disease squeezing vitality from their faces. Some women are considered gorgeous in the world's eyes, movie-star worthy and worshipped for their high cheek bones and outward physique. Some are teased as the ugly duckling, downgraded as unimportant by the world's standards and narcissistic vanity; some are seen as misfits by society—but never by our infinite Creator.

Certainly, each person is different. And some of us have diseases or disabilities, and the Heavenly Potter has allowed it.

> *"But now, O Lord, You are our Father; we are the clay, and You our*
> *potter; and all of us are the work of Your hand."*
> – Isaiah 64:8

But our God is the Father of good gifts.

> *"Every good thing given and every perfect gift is from above, coming*
> *down from the Father of lights, with whom there is no variation*
> *or shifting shadow."*
> – James 1:17

He delights in us, and we are His children; never let anyone tell you otherwise. The world is wrong! Christ Himself was not pretty of form and face.

> *"For He grew up before Him like a tender shoot, and like a root out of*
> *parched ground; He has no stately form or majesty that we should*
> *look upon Him, nor appearance that we should be attracted to Him."*
> – Isaiah 53:2

You are created by the One who uses the poor, despised, and shamed of the world to make a difference, to further the Gospel for His kingdom. He looks at the heart.

> *"But the LORD said to Samuel, 'Do not look at his appearance*
> *or at the height of his stature, because I have rejected him;*

for God sees not as man sees, for man looks at the outward appear-
ance, but the Lord looks at the heart'."
– 1 Samuel 16:7

Therefore, we were made on purpose, and we bear disease because the earth fell into sin when Adam and Eve chose disobedience and the Lord allowed the effects of the Fall. These effects have an impact on our bodies, our vegetation, and the earth on which we labor, toil, and strive.

Physically, this disease can affect us, but spiritually, we should not pretend to let it touch us. Instead, through Him, we can let this disease or disability change us for His good. It can make us powerhouse Christian women: women who are stronger, kinder, and more patient; women who have more faith, who are obedient to His Word and trust in His plan; women who know the power of God's Word in their lives and will be there for others, to comfort, encourage, and spur them on. It's our spiritual heart, not our physical heart, that should concern us; we should be focused on how we can use our hearts of faith to bring God the highest Honor to His esteemed name. Our heartbeat for Christ will not die when we die physically but will beat in eternity forevermore. Our whole heart should be used to pulsate for the One who originated it before He spoke the world into existence. We can have a Christ-like storehouse that, spiritually, is not affected by disease.

With Your counsel You will guide me,
And afterward receive me to glory.
Whom have I in heaven but You?
And besides You, I desire nothing on earth.
My flesh and my heart may fail,
But God is the strength of my heart and my portion forever.
– Psalm 73:24-26

He created our heart; He knows we're enduring disability or disease. Instead of us dreading life, God calls us to be content, trusting in Him, even if our bodies are like stale bread that crumbles at the touch. He can use this trial and gift of disease to make us resemble Him more and more. Without His unfailing love and without Him creating us, we would not be here. He is our Creator.

THE EARTH IS THE LORD'S

"The earth is the Lord's, and all it contains, the world, and those who dwell in it" (Psalm 24:1). We see from this verse that our Abba Father owns everything, and since we live on earth, we can see once again that we belong to Him. God not only created us, making Him our Father, our Creator, but the earth is His as well. He is the rightful owner. He owns it as well as all of us. The Bible says no one is excused. People don't want to acknowledge that God created them and that He is their rightful owner. Man wants to belong to himself and not have to answer to anyone, so that he can indulge in his sin. Men and women denying God have hardened their hearts; they have set themselves up as their own God, and that's why they suppress the Truth.

For the wrath of God is revealed from heaven against all ungodliness and unrighteousness of men who suppress the truth in unrighteousness, because that which is known about God is evident within them; for God made it evident to them. For since the creation of the world His invisible attributes, His eternal power and divine nature, have been clearly seen, being understood through what has been made, so that they are without excuse. For even though they knew God, they did not honor Him as God or give thanks, but they became futile in their speculations, and their foolish heart was darkened. Professing to be wise, they became fools, and exchanged the glory of the incorruptible God for an image in the form of corruptible man and of birds and four-footed animals and crawling creatures (Romans 1:18-23).

But one day, unsaved mankind will have to answer as to why they rejected Christ and strived to seek their own god, whether that be the god of pleasure, money, pride, or deceit, and they will have to answer for every immoral deed, thought, and act they committed.

GOD IS HOLY

"... *it is written, 'You shall be holy, for I am holy,'*" (1 Peter 1:16). If you've been in church at all, opened a Bible, or listened to Christian music, I'm sure you've heard the term holy. God is holy. Holy means pure and without sin; He is to be revered. So, since we understand that we're created by God and that He is over all, we need to also understand that God is holy. Our God is a Holy Creator, a Holy God. He owns every breath, every step, every personal disease or disability that affects us. He owns our smiles, tears, days, years, and burdens, as well as all the tender mirth of life we experience. He sews us together like a patchwork quilt, full of colorful squares, big and small. Each person, each "quilt" in this entire universe, He makes differently but sews them all in completeness. My quilt, my life, has been threaded to express His plan for me. Each quilt becomes a tapestry of our faith, our soul covering, if you will, and as devout followers, we are sewn together into one large mosaic of squares on end; we are all part of His plan if you are His.

God is perfect, flawless, without blemish, without sin. *"You know that He appeared in order to take away sins; and in Him there is no sin"* (1 John 3:5).

As such, He cannot even look upon sin. "*Your* eyes are too pure to approve evil, *and You cannot look on wickedness with favor*" (Habakkuk 1:13).

As human beings, sin is rampant and coerces our thoughts, motives, actions, decisions, and conversations; it's uncontainable. The world serves it up on a big ladle and feeds it to us disguised as Mary Poppins' sparkly concoction. The voice of Satan, the serpent's hissing drawl, whispers hypnotically, "Just a spoon full of sugar helps the medicine go down," and it easily drenches our ever-parched throat. Sin lives in every human being. We swallow its sugary syrup, addicted to the world's poison, never knowing the cyanide soaking in. We have soggy souls without Christ, and we're being eaten from the inside out without even realizing it. Women can work out, take supplements, cook Paleo, use their juicers every morning, make kabocha smoothies, and buy organic everything at the grocery store, but if their minds and hearts have not been fed the Living Word, the poison is corroding their lost soul, and they are only physically fit, not soul fit. Sin is poison. We are addicted to sin; it's our choice drug. Sin is the demise of Veruca Salt in *Charlie and the Chocolate Factory* (1971 film).

"I want it now!" she barks, then stands on the scale to weigh the golden eggs, and down the garbage chute she goes, along with all the other bad eggs. *We* are the bad eggs without Christ.

We sin not only against others, but we sin against our Holy Father. We sin against our Sovereign in so many ways. We do not acknowledge Him or His laws when we're plotting out how to sin or committing a sin we're not admitting. We choose to ignore His commands, proving that committing our sin is more important to us than the Holy of Holies. We can be hypocrites as we look down on others, indulging heavily in their same sin when no one is looking. We can let our disease become our favorite idol as we choose to drown in it instead of swimming to the shores of God's grace and His Word.

So how can the verse, 1 Peter 1:16, say "be holy"? How does God expect people to "be holy as I am holy"? How does the Lord of Creation expect us to be perfect when we're submerged in sin and imperfection? God is the only One who can be faultless . . . yet God is saying that He requires untainted obedience from us, for us to be defect-less.

"Therefore, you are to be perfect as your heavenly Father is perfect."
– Matthew 5:48

So how do we do that? How is that possible? This verse begins with "therefore," meaning He has put the responsibility on us. But I can look at myself and know that I am the furthest thing from "stainless," and for any human it's an impossible measure to attain. I get angry, I've lied, I've stolen, I've coveted; people commit these kinds of acts every day. I've been downcast, hidden in darkness, trying to wish away my disease to no avail, and in my fleshly, angry heart, I've seen my Lord as a mean, unfair genie who refuses to come out of the lamp, grant my three wishes, and poof!—make my disease disappear. We're all guilty of being unholy. Perfect people don't mess up. They don't do these things.

The Bible calls these "sins" and says that when we sin, we break His law. Sin is "to miss the mark" and signifies the trespass or transgression of law. So, man is sinful. Man misses the mark and the standard of perfection. We can't even begin to pick up a bow and arrow and hit the bull's-eye; it's like we're blindfolded, spun around 100 times, and then told to shoot the arrow and have it land dead center, not even a tiny bit off to the left or right. We'll miss the mark every time. This is man before salvation. Man is guilty. Man is guilty of breaking God's law, man is not holy, man has nothing to offer, and man is sinful and corrupt throughout, falling short of God's standard.

> *"For all have sinned and fall short of the glory of God."*
> – Romans 3:23

> *"For whoever keeps the whole law and yet stumbles in one point he has become guilty of all."*
> – James 2:10

These verses tell us that man cannot keep the law; we all fall short of God's glory. If you've committed sin just once in your life—lied, expressed and/or acted in unrighteous anger, been covetous, sped on the highway, been without hope and buried in bitterness because of your disease, worrisome, anxious, even thinking a bad thought—then you're a lawbreaker. There's a "WANTED" sign on your back, with a reward if you're caught; you're a criminal. You've transgressed and must serve time for your crime. You've sinned by breaking God's law; the sheriff is in town to lock you up and throw away the key, declaring "You are guilty!" We're all guilty because, once more, *"All have sinned and fall short of the glory God"* (Romans 3:23).

So again, the question is this: how can we be whole and blameless? How can we meet God's standard of living a sin-free life? We've all sinned against God. We're not innocent, and there are consequences for sin. Our consequence? That we deserve eternal punishment, that we deserve death. We deserve to be in Hell because we broke God's law.

> *"Everyone who practices sin also practices lawlessness; and sin is lawlessness."*
> – 1 John 3:4

In a courtroom, when someone is guilty, the judge bangs the gavel and sentences the person. The guilty must pay for the crime and be sentenced. Why? Because they broke the law. Justice tells us that the crime must be paid for, and since we sin and break God's law, we must be sentenced. Death is our earned outcome. Because we sin, there's not only physical death but eternal death and separation from Christ that we will face.

"He who believes in the Son has eternal life; but he who does not obey the Son will not see life, but the wrath of God abides on him."

– John 3:36

This verse also sums it up well:

Otherwise, He [Jesus] would have needed to suffer often since the foundation of the world; but now once at the consummation of the ages He has been manifested to put away sin by the sacrifice of Himself. And in as much as it is appointed for men to die once and after this comes judgment.

– Hebrews 9:26-27

The Bible tells us, *"For the wages of sin is death but the gift of God is eternal life in Christ Jesus our Lord"* (Romans 6:23). This is where the Good News comes in, the celebration, the clapping of hands and loud cheering applause for His radical and purposeful remedy of sin. He offers a sacrifice, paying for our sin in full.

JESUS IS OUR SACRIFICE

"For God so loved the world, that He gave His only begotten Son, that whoever believes in Him shall not perish, but have eternal life."

– John 3:16

God sent His Son, Jesus Christ. Don't you just feel a smile come to your face, don't you just want to drop to your knees, prostrate in worship, imagining the gift that He imputed to us as sinners—because Jesus, the King of the Jews, chose to put on our sin? Adam, the first man, disobeyed Man's Maker, and we live as fallen beings because of his choice.

> *Therefore, just as through one man sin entered into the world, and death through sin, and so death spread to all men, because all sinned—for until the Law sin was in the world, but sin is not imputed when there is no law. Nevertheless, death reigned from Adam until Moses, even over those who had not sinned in the likeness of the offense of Adam, who is a type of Him who was to come.*
> *But the free gift is not like the transgression. For if by the transgression of the one the many died, much more did the grace of God and the gift by the grace of the one Man, Jesus Christ, abound to the many.*
> – Romans 5:12-15

Christ was our grace that abounded because of the Father's love. *"But God demonstrates His own love toward us, in that while we were yet sinners, Christ died for us"* (Romans 5:8), and *"He made Him who knew no sin to be sin on our behalf, so that we might become the righteousness of God in Him"* (2 Corinthians 5:21).

Because someone had to pay the penalty for sin, sin had to be dealt with by someone who was holy and perfect, who was flesh and blood, just like you and me but without sin. Jesus paid the price for our sins. Jesus was the one because Jesus is God in the flesh. Jesus was our substitute.

I love the old hymn that sings, "The vilest offender who truly believes, that moment from Jesus a pardon receives, is our freedom song. This is the gift. The free, no strings attached, costless, liberating gift." There is nothing we've done to earn our salvation; as many of the Scripture verses in this chapter state, we are sinful and need to be saved from eternal death. God gives us this gift through His only Son, Jesus Christ, who shed His blood and laid down His life; the Father sacrificed His Son in our place. Jesus died for you. He stood in your place. As the impeccable substitute, He died for all the sins you would ever commit, past, present and future. The Lamb Who Takes Away the Sin of the World was condemned, sheered, and led to the cross, slain bloody and gory, without an ounce of remorse or sadness from us or from the ones who first welcomed Him to this godless world, who then sold him out for Barabbas, a guilty thief and murderer.

"But you disowned the Holy and Righteous One and asked for a murderer to be granted to you."

– Acts 3:14

"But they cried out all together, saying, 'Away with this man, and release for us Barabbas!'"

– Luke 23:18

BUT YOU ARE SAVED BY . . .

. . . Calling on the name of the Lord! *". . . for whoever will call on the name of the Lord will be saved"* (Romans 10:13).

Salvation is that simple: salvation is for anyone who receives Christ as her Lord and Savior. You don't have to have a mansion in the wealthy part of town; a penniless beggar in a back alleyway has just as much hope in being saved. You don't have to be a certain physical stature and able to enter a marathon; you can be crippled and permanently disabled in a wheelchair. You don't have to be a religious theologian; you can have opened your Bible for the first time and read the Gospel. You can be a seven-year-old at your mother's knee or a ninety-year-old in a nursing home, about to slip from this life. You can be a thief like Barabbas or a murderer like Herod, or you could have been brought up in the church squeaky clean. Just understand that Jesus is the only way to God.

"Jesus said to him, 'I am the way, and the truth, and the life; no one comes to the Father but through Me'."

– John 14:6

He is the only path to eternal life. Following other gods won't give you salvation—not Buddha, not Mormonism's Joseph Smith with the gold plates, not Muhammad and Allah of Islam, not Gandhi and the gods of Hindus, not the good works of Catholicism, not mysticism, not Scientology, not New Age philosophy, not reincarnation. Saving faith lies in Christ alone. Salvation is believing and repenting of your sin, and it's believing that God the Father allowed His Son to be killed in your place. It's believing Jesus is God in the flesh, the innocent for the guilty, that He died on the cross, and on the third day later, rose from the dead, sitting today in heaven at the Father's right hand.

If you believe that Jesus is your Lord and Savior and paid for your sin, and you receive salvation as a gift and put your faith and your trust in Him, and if you know you are a sinner and have confessed and prayed to the Lord and have repented—turned from your old way of life, your sin, and want to live for Christ—you are saved.

I will see you one day. We are forever sisters who will worship the Lord in His beaconed refulgence.

So, bow your head and repent. He may be drawing you to His side right now. The disease you thought was a curse could be how He causes you to surrender your life to Him. Find someone you know as a Christian, and if you have questions, ask him or her. Repent and believe in Christ and receive salvation!

THE BEAUTIFUL AND AGONIZING TRUTH

The truth is both beautiful and agonizing: the battle you're fighting because of your illness lies in the hands that were pierced with nails. Jesus understands the sorrow, pain, and physical suffering you and I face and sweat through daily. He did not have a disease or disability, but His sorrow, His agonizing pain, was far more serious. Not only was He crucified and tortured, but unlike us, He also experienced the spiritual departure and abandonment of God, His Father who watched Him take on sin and bodily torture without lifting His hand to stop it.

He trusts in God; Let God rescue Him now, if he delights in Him; for He said, "I am the Son of God." The robbers who had been crucified with Him were also insulting Him with the same words.

> *Now from the sixth hour darkness fell upon all the land until the ninth hour. About the ninth hour Jesus cried out with a loud voice, saying, "Eli, Eli, lama sabachthani?" that is, "My God, My God, why have You forsaken Me?" And some of those who were standing there, when they heard it, began saying, "This man is calling for Elijah." Immediately one of them ran, and taking a sponge, he filled it with sour wine and put it on a reed, and gave Him a drink. But the rest of them said, "Let us see whether Elijah will come to save Him." And Jesus cried out again with a loud voice, and yielded up His spirit.*
> – Matthew 27:43-50

Friends, our Jesus, the God-man, felt pain. He felt the nails that held up His body until the full and sweltering wrath of our awesome God unleashed every sin on Him, and He bore it willingly.

*"For Christ also died for sins once for all, the just for the unjust, so
that He might bring us to God, having been put to death in the flesh,
but made alive in the spirit."*
– 1 Peter 3:18

He bore the curse we left on the world, so we could have peace
and restitution with our Maker. He sacrificed His sacred life for our
tarnished and rusted soul—His righteousness traded for our sins. He
gave us His glory and was paraded in our defeat: His cloak of light for
our dingy, dusty, filthy rags. God wants us to know that when we repent, then all the sins we've committed, past, present, and future—our
daily physical transgressions, our former man, the struggle with our
flesh in the midst of the trials of our disease or disability—is still a
constant battle, but our life is secure in Christ. God's will was fulfilled
by treating Christ the way He should have treated you and me. "It is
finished!" cried out Christ on the cross.

*"Therefore, when Jesus had received the sour wine, He said, 'It is fin-
ished!' And He bowed His head and gave up His spirit."*
– John 19:30

Indeed, it was finished; it has been accomplished, His death for
our new life.

BUTTERFLY IN THE SKY

Some of you may have handicaps or bones and joints that swell and
deform, and some reading this may have endured the pain of looking
vastly different in face and figure because of how disease is affecting
your physical body. Perhaps your medication and the effects of surgeries make you feel like your health is peeling away, just as the skin falls

off a ripe banana. Some of you brush your paper-thin hair and watch it fall to the floor like scattered party confetti, and some of you now wear a wig to cover your shiny bald head; your once-long locks have succumbed to the radiation or the side effects of prescription drugs.

Maybe you're dealing with the dreaded "moon face," as some women nickname it, because you have puffy cheeks, the steroids taking their toll. Other women are resembling walking skeletons, with flesh now gone, bones protruding, and skin "freckled purple" from head toe, the tell-tale bruises left from repeated shots and blood transfusions. My friend, if you feel and see your body rotting away like a decaying tree limb desperate for the rain, please know you're not alone!

Other women, too, are sitting in hospital chairs nauseated, the chemo-like viper's venom swimming through their bloodstream, flowing to every part of their body; they try to stay calm as they make uneasy chatter with the administering nurse. Some women with disease are putting on their best poker face, without emotion, and you'd never know that inside they're screaming at the top of their lungs while feeling their compromised body shutting down. Some of you are poked and prodded with needles; others continue to throw up because of harsh side effects of medicine from the latest doctor trying to cure you; and some of you who must keep getting infusion after infusion, painfully and repeatedly, are feeling like a factory belt in an assembly line that just keeps running.

But you are also His child, and He is with you. He assures us we will rise one day on the wings of eagles. *"Yet those who wait for the Lord will gain new strength; they will mount up with wings like eagles, they will run and not get tired, they will walk and not become weary"* (Isaiah 40:31).

We can hope in the truth of that day coming because our physical body is not where we place our hope; it can fail us daily. Rather, our hope stands firmly, resolutely in the Lord.

> *Many are saying of my soul,*
> *"There is no deliverance for him in God."*
> *But You, O Lord, are a shield about me,*
> *My glory, and the One who lifts my head.*
> *I was crying to the Lord with my voice,*
> *And He answered me from His holy mountain.*
> *I lay down and slept;*
> *I awoke, for the Lord sustains me.*
>
> – Psalm 3:2-5

YOUR HIGHNESS

Young teenage girls with disease reading this, please know: when you walk down your school hallways or are pushed in a wheelchair to classes, as you go to the park, grocery store, or mall if you're able, as you go to one more doctor appointment or sit in your buttoned-up hospital gown with curtains drawn in your shaded room, the standard, big floral picture on the wall to your right and the fake leather visitor's chair to the side, and if perhaps you feel ugly because of your disease or disability, please know that you are God's elected royalty. Trusting in Jesus for your salvation, you're a chosen child, Christ's coheir, His most precious design, and though you may be physically sick or disabled, you're spiritually already healed.

Your godly character is being displayed by the countenance you wear on your face; by the pursed smile on your gaunt cheeks; by the love you speak to others through a good God always with you; by the joy that only those who know Christ can understand and that proves so contagious in your words and actions! So, hold your cute, mighty head up high so your invisible tiara won't slip, and if it does, push it right back up, and all those jewels and precious stones adorning it will say who you are: an exquisite gem, a sparkling diadem. You are *magnifique*, as they say in France.

God doesn't do ugly; His creations always exude grace and impeccable glamour. So, let it make you a role-model for the Gospel at your school and with your friends. By showing the trust you have in Christ, you can be a testimony of Truth in a warped generation and not consumed with popularity, who's dating who, or the latest phone app. Instead, choose to be excellent in character. Remember, we should model His life:

> But you did not learn Christ in this way, if indeed you have heard Him
> and have been taught in Him, just as truth is in Jesus, that, in refer-
> ence to your former manner of life, you lay aside the old self, which
> is being corrupted in accordance with the lusts of deceit, and that
> you be renewed in the spirit of your mind, and put on the new self,
> which in the likeness of God has been created in righteousness and
> holiness of the truth.
> – Ephesians 4:20-24

As saved sisters, our Creator made us a new creation when He opened our eyes through the work of the Spirit and gave us His salvation. When we become Christians, with or without disease, we're a "new man."

When Clark Kent goes into a telephone booth, he becomes Superman, a new man with supernatural powers, but Superman must become his old self once more, just another news reporter and no longer the red-caped guy with the snazzy gold *S* on his chest, flying through the sky and saving the day. Superman may slip off his new self at will, but as Christ-followers, we never do; we are always a new creation.

Paul never became Saul again, a stop-at-nothing persecutor of the church, set on seeking out Christians to rid the world of the beliefs they held true. The woman at the well, whole and pure, a bride fit to walk down the aisle for the King of kings, never returned to her adulterous ways. The centurion was never again under Roman authority, but followed only his new Commander, the Lord who commands the heavenly hosts and who will break the seals one day. The thief on the cross was no longer a chained-up heart about to face the eternal fire of Satan's lair, but a free, new man sailing the crystal-clear water, with the wind catching the coastal breeze and guiding him across the banks of the Jordan into the paradise guaranteed by his Lord. Mary Magdalene was no longer demon possessed but out of spiritual bondage. The woman who broke the oil and anointed Christ no longer mocked and taunted, no longer made her living at night in the disguise of the dark, but was cleansed and saved, being made new as she anointed the Anointed One.

I'm always a new creation in Christ. You're always a new creation in Christ. Disease and disability do not take that from us. We are gorgeous, like butterflies spreading our technicolor wings as we come upon a glossy gale and take to the grace-filled sky. So, flutter your wings and begin to fly. Soar as a free creature; the bumpy, lumpy, pokey caterpillar is gone and is now a supernatural, beauteous butterfly taking the world by storm, cocoon far behind and now looking ahead and soaring free. The old is gone; you are new!

"Therefore if anyone is in Christ, he is a new creature; the old things passed away; behold, new things have come."

– 2 Corinthians 5:17

IS DISEASE STEALING YOUR JOY?

So beloved sisters, think about how sin can impact you with your disease and disability. Think about all the ways we let sin steal our joy. When we doubt God's goodness because of our disease, it's called sin. Instead of reeling in doubt, we should know He is good.

"The Lord is good to all, and His mercy is over all His works."

– Psalm 145:9

When we're not content with where He has us in our life, blaming our attitude on our disease, we're acting sinfully. The Lord shows us that our contentment is not based on who we are, what kind of disease we have, and if a cure is found; our contentment isn't rooted in *if* we have a roof over our head, clothes on our back, or even know from where our next meal will come. Contentment is lived out as we no longer worry nor fret over each day, each breath, each doctor appointment, as we no longer see our pulse quicken nor our mind swirl with thoughts of doubt like the silver McDonald's machine churning out ice cream. Instead, turn your mind and heart to your Heavenly Father, and ask Him to let your mind rest on Truth.

*Therefore, I tell you, do not worry about your life, what you will
eat or drink; or about your body, what you will wear. Is not life
more than food, and the body more than clothes? Look at the birds
of the air; they do not sow or reap or store away in barns, and yet
your heavenly Father feeds them. Are you not much more valuable
than they?*

– Matthew 6:25-26

When anger rears its ugly, sinful head because someone who doesn't understand what we go through made a comment—or when we awake in the morning at times disgruntled and depressed to start the day—we're in sin. When God doesn't physically heal us, but we expect Him to do so and get anxious and start doubting He cares, we sin. When we see someone, someone we love diagnosed or living with disease or disability and we question God, we are sinning. When those around us are without disease and we envy them, or when we worry what the future will bring because the hospital visit is full of shocking news and we want to blame God, this is sin.

When the physical pain is daunting, and you think, "Why me?" and question His love and care, or when the radiation is eating away at your body and you start to let it eat away at your soul, and on and on, those are all sins. You see, sisters, we have all sinned, and the war with sin is never over. But Christ took those sins and removed them from us a distance stretching into infinity.

"As far as the east is from the west, so far has He removed our trans-gressions from us."

– Psalm 103:12

We've all thought bad thoughts, become frustrated, been angry with someone, been envious, and at times even lost hope because of disease. Those sins that you and I continually contend with, that sometimes follow us into the night, that question God and ask, "Why me?"—they are wrong.

When we think to ourselves, "Why am I the one who carries with me the crushing weight of this disease day in and day out?" or "Why am I the one who wakes each morning knowing I'll again face the same relentless anguish I faced yesterday?," please know that those sins are washed away in the light of His work on the cross when you repent of them. Amen! Had Christ not become a man who lifted the curse and gave mankind reconciliation to God the Father, we would still be walking around dead in our sin and trespasses, no hope in sight. We'd still be stumbling in the dark, in blindness, without God and without Christ, destined for Hell, and still living with a physical disease or disability. But the good and great news is that when we repent of those sins, we're washed perfectly white and flawlessly spotless.

"Purify me with hyssop, and I shall be clean; wash me, and I shall
be whiter than snow."

– Psalm 51:7

If you're not in Christ as you're reading this book's early pages, I pray you're asking yourself, "So how can I be saved?"

The simple answer is "by believing the Gospel."

It's that easy—salvation is a gift, free and clear.

"Why Christ?" you might be wondering. Because He never committed a sin; He was perfect. Christ was perfect in word, thought, and deed, and He fully obeyed God's plan actively in His obedience and passively in His suffering. Yes, He was willing to suffer immensely. He was sacrificed, His holy body given for our grotesque sin, and His undefiled blood was drained for you and me.

If you believe that Jesus is God, that He died and was raised and sits at the Father's right hand, if you believe He is the Way, and you repent of your sin and make Him Lord and Master of your life, then you have salvation. These key verses confirm this amazing truth:

. . . fixing our eyes on Jesus, the author and perfecter of faith, who for
the joy set before Him endured the cross, despising the shame, and
has sat down at the right hand of the throne of God.

– Hebrews 12:2

Jesus said to him, "I am the way, and the truth, and the life; no one comes to the Father but through Me."
– John 14:6

OUR ANCHOR

I want to pause for a second and pose another question. Whatever you're going through with disease or disability—whether you're daily battling its wretched attacks on your body, whether you're watching and caring for someone you love endure that exhausting struggle, or whether you're grieving a deeply treasured person on this earth who's lost the earthly battle and memories are persistently welling up in your heart each time you see his or her face in a photograph, ones you'll now never remove from the frame—can you imagine the kind of depression and recurrent hopelessness someone experiences without faith in Christ? Can you imagine that kind of sadness and loneliness? Just think about fighting this battle without salvation and without Jesus as your Anchor, who quells the waves of life as they thrust upon you. Imagine your life without Jesus, with the doubt, struggle, and sin ruling your life with no way to stop them. Can you feel the emptiness when there's no one to turn to, no hope, no certainty of eternal life in heaven?

I pray you don't know that kind of emptiness. I pray you do not know the wrath of God when you die. Do you feel those waves in aggression tearing apart your sails and trying to drown you in misery, not relinquishing but forcing you farther and farther out into exposed waters?

Jesus, our great Sacrifice, is the Anchor that holds our souls and keeps the storms we face at bay, which threaten to pelt down on our ever-fragile hearts.

"This hope we have as an anchor of the soul, a hope both sure and
steadfast and one which enters within the veil."
– Hebrews 6:19

He is our Anchor and our Promise that has already come to pass; He is our salvation. We have a right standing, a clean slate, an innocent verdict in God's courtroom. Case dismissed! Hallelujah, that's a jubilant truth.

So, what can we learn on this journey of bearing disease?

First, understand that God offers us His Chronic Love that gives us salvation. No matter what you face, you face it with security. People without Christ have empty hearts, dead and hardened.

"... being darkened in their understanding, excluded from the life of
God because of the ignorance that is in them, because of the hard-
ness of their heart."
– Ephesians 4:18

I know this because, before Christ, that described me. I can remember that all the material pleasures, friends, and love from others were never enough. I was never satisfied. I would wake up in the morning with that same uncomfortable pang stabbing my heart, sticking in the side of my soul like a pointy splinter, which couldn't be removed. The sin I committed ruled my life, and while I took pleasure in it for a moment, the sullen emptiness was always there. Sin didn't satisfy fully my hunger but only left me wanting more. The more I sinned, the quicker my steps fell on the steep path that would lead me to destruction.

The uneasiness of not knowing what could happen without my earthly comforts—and even those comforts themselves—left me asking, "Is this it?" In college, I was saved through faith in Christ, and I married while in college, but then like a time bomb, my disease exploded and took over my body; there were and still are daily times of physical, and spiritual battles, but praise be to God, I have Christ. I have eternal life! I have a Savior who died for me.

Where does your comfort come from? Your eternal security? Your peace and strength in having a disease? If you are not in *Christ*, none exist! You can try to rationalize and philosophize; you can be a genius, millionaire, successful business woman, or put-together PTA mom. You can possess all the worldly treasures; go to church every Sunday; be the humanitarian that cures social injustice and fights for human rights; or be the girl who thinks her outside looks determine her inner worth. You can be a hero in society's eyes, serve at the soup kitchen every Friday like clockwork, even be on the women's leadership team at your church. But, if you haven't received Christ as your Lord and Savior, then all your good works are like filthy rags, and the path you're on will lead you astray and end in death.

> *"For all of us have become like one who is unclean, and all our righteous deeds are like a filthy garment; and all of us wither like a leaf, and our iniquities, like the wind, take us away."*
> – Isaiah 64:6

The Bible talks about it being a narrow door that will be shut to those who cannot enter the skinny way.

> *And someone said to Him, "Lord, are there just a few who are being saved?" And He said to them, "Strive to enter through the narrow door; for many, I tell you, will seek to enter and will not be able. Once the head of the house gets up and shuts the door, and you begin to stand*

outside and knock on the door, saying, 'Lord, open up to us!' then He
will answer and say to you, 'I do not know where you are from.'"
– Luke 13:23-25

There is no faith without Christ, no eternal rest promised; and without Christ, any loyal love is only a hollow, stony muscle in your chest. But if you have salvation, God gives you a new heart.

"Moreover, I will give you a new heart and put a new spirit within
you; and I will remove the heart of stone from your flesh and give
you a heart of flesh."
– Ezekiel 36:26

Beloved sister, disease without Christ is letting the disease win. It's like letting your life go to waste and being tossed in the landfill, and then after you die without Christ, an eternity of even worse begins . . .

But life with Christ is being alive. Heavenly freedom feels like Paul and Silas breaking out of their chains, busting open the doors of their jail cell and crying out to their God in esteemed worship for rescuing them. It's truly taking a breath without breathing in polluted air. The person receiving Christ is like a weight no one can lift being hoisted and snapped in two like a wishbone. Life with Christ is unending joy, bubbling over like a babbling brook on a country mountainside. Life in Him is coming alive after being dead. His rescuing is the feeling of riding in a fiery red, smooth convertible with the top down, feeling the swift breeze racing through your hair while singing praise songs at the top of your lungs. It's Him breathing new life into your cold-corpse soul, opening the coffin of your old you and stepping out into the new name you're now called: Forgiven!

This is our life with Christ; and with disease or disability, we need Him to carry us in His strength through our impossible-in-ourselves-but-capable-through-Him trials. This is how you should lay your head down at night, knowing peace and protection, knowing we have a future to look to just ahead. He gives spiritual life, He gives spiritual blessings, and He never, ever stops loving you. He is a faithful God, and your soul can never be snatched away. There is no disease or disability, no matter how crushing or devastating, that can sever you spiritually if you're in Christ, not even death.

> *For I am convinced that neither death, nor life, nor angels, nor principalities, nor things present, nor things to come, nor powers, nor height, nor depth, nor any other created thing, will be able to separate us from the love of God, which is in Christ Jesus our Lord.*
>
> – Romans 8:38-39

The Bible is about the old becoming new, the sick being healed, the imprisoned made free. The Bible is about those healed spiritually and some even healed both physically and spiritually. It's an Index of Hope. You're included if you're saved and you're a brand-new creation just like those in Scripture, on whom He set His love by drawing them to Him as the Holy Spirit wooed. He has set Himself up in our hearts to change us, to give us supernatural viability by drawing us to Him through the Gospel.

> *"No one can come to Me unless the Father who sent Me draws him; and I will raise him up on the last day."*
>
> – John 6:44

You are His prized, gold star possession, like when a child draws her first picture of herself and sees a simple stick figure while God sees a sensational masterpiece, more exquisite than a Michelangelo rarity. You are the first-picked, juicy red apple of His eye. Don't let your disease make you live as the old "man," causing you to give in to sin. Fight sin because we're no longer under its power and control. We can live in the trust of our Lord and what He has for us each moment of each day. If each day is filled with suffering, then each day will be filled with promise and faith—all the help from Him we need to sustain us—giving us that supernatural ability to live with disease.

YOU ARE NOT ALONE

We are not the only ones who feel pain. Pain was also felt by Christ as He hung on the cross. We're never alone in the anguish we feel. Never. Our salvation was a gift to us, but for Christ it cost Him His life. It was weighty, and He was buried and rose on the third day from the tomb. You have suffering because of disease, but when you're enduring it, remember you have a Best Friend in Christ, a Brother who was a sacrifice, beaten, tortured, whipped, and forced to carry His own cross (before God enlisted Simon of Cyrene to help shoulder it to Golgotha). He was denied three times by Peter, one of His closest disciples, and was betrayed by a kiss from Judas, another chosen disciple. Christ suffered unjustly, but He used His last breath to utter life and victory for you, not to cry for help but to assure His children that He had broken sin's curse and had given us New Life and forgiveness of sins past, present, and future, if we have repentant hearts.

THE SUFFERING SERVANT

We can understand that when we doubt, we can keep our countenance holy and pure. When the pain is inadmissible, and we sin in word, thought, or deed, succumbing to the heartaches disease can bring, we know we're forgiven as our hearts our washed in Christ's atoning sacrifice. For me, having an always-present disease can bring gnawing pain, drowning fatigue, continual doubt, and looming uncertainty in what my future will be like. I ask questions such as, "Will I even be here to see my daughter grow up and get married and begin her adult life?"

Yet, when I lift up my eyes to Christ, and repent of my sin, all those thoughts and doubts are erased, and I'm assured of my relationship with Him. I can face pain, mocking, ridicule, even torture, if He calls me to do so. He felt pain—sovereignly, faithfully—and He died so our souls would never feel the separation of not being with Him. Physical pain may ail us in this life, but it will vanish like a vapor in the next. Reflect on His pain; reflect on His suffering. He did not let you face this disease or disability without facing torture Himself:

> Then the soldiers of the governor took Jesus into the Praetorium and gathered the whole Roman cohort around Him. They stripped Him and put a scarlet robe on Him. And after twisting together a crown of thorns, they put it on His head, and a reed in His right hand; and they knelt down before Him and mocked Him, saying, "Hail, King of the Jews!" They spat on Him, and took the reed and began to beat Him on the head. After they had mocked Him, they took the scarlet robe off Him and put His own garments back on Him, and led Him away to crucify Him.
>
> – Matthew 27:27-31

You ache and hurt at times, and He knows that pain as He was tortured; He hurt and He ached. His example is there for you to glean a proper perspective and a biblical framework. I cannot ever say, "Well, He doesn't know what physical pain feels like," or "He's never gone through it," because He has.

> *He was despised and forsaken of men,*
> *A man of sorrows and acquainted with grief;*
> *And like one from whom men hide their face*
> *He was despised, and we did not esteem Him.*
> *Surely our griefs He Himself bore,*
> *And our sorrows He carried;*
> *Yet we ourselves esteemed Him stricken,*
> *Smitten of God, and afflicted.*
> *But He was pierced through for our transgressions,*
> *He was crushed for our iniquities;*
> *The chastening for our well-being fell upon Him,*
> *And by His scourging we are healed.*
>
> – Isaiah 53:3-5

We are loved by the One who suffered as well. God the Father gave His Son, and Christ watched His Father ignore His merciful cries; He watched Him look away and be pleased to crush Him.

> *"But the Lord was pleased to crush Him, putting Him to grief; If He would render Himself as a guilt offering, He will see His offspring, He will prolong His days, and the good pleasure of the Lord will prosper in His hand."*
>
> – Isaiah 53:10

Christ knows dejection, grief, a broken heart, and physical, wretched woe and sorrow. He knows what you're living with, dealing with, struggling with. He knows who you are with your disease or disability as a caregiver as well. And His Word calls us to boast in His name.

> *"Some boast in chariots and some in horses, but we will boast in the*
> *name of the Lord, our God."*
>
> – Psalm 20:7

Trust the Lord with your pain and the plan He has for you. Morning and night, cling to Jesus, the Suffering Servant and His Word, and know He is your salvation, your Chronic Savior.

> "If man had his way, the plan of redemption would be an endless and bloody conflict. Salvation was bought not by Jesus' fist, but by His nail-pierced hands; not by muscle but by love; not by vengeance but by forgiveness; not by force but by sacrifice. Jesus Christ our Lord surrendered in order that He might win; He destroyed His enemies by dying for them and conquered death by allowing death to conquer Him."
>
> – A.W. Tozer, *Preparing for Jesus' Return: Daily Live the*
> *Blessed Hope*[1]

CHRIST THE LADDER

When you think about facing this disease and the pain and suffering that come with it, know each day you must prepare your mind to keep taking steps, an ability fueled in how you see your disease. Using the illustration of a ladder can help! Think of Christ as your Ladder, and continue climbing up, trusting that He won't break, and knowing He'll hold you steady as you climb. And when you face the depressed times because of your disease or disability, know that one day you'll see the

---

1 Tozer, A.W. *Preparing for Jesus' Return: Daily Live the Blessed Hope.* Bloomington: Bethany House Publishers. 2012.

Son light. He is light; He is the Bright and Morning Star, the true Son Light. Don't view your disease as darkness, a black hole, a doomed pit. Look up, see the ladder, and use it to climb out of your misery—each rung, step by step, inching you a little closer to the rays of light streaming in. Christ is your Ladder! Our God, our Christ, is steady. He will hold you up. If you're in Him, there's nothing that can pull you off that Ladder. Trust in Him, trust in His salvation, the only way that leads to eternal life. Rejoice! You have salvation; your heart is owned and kept by the Everlasting One, our Awesome Abba, the One who will one day take away your disease or disability forever. Never again will it plague you, causing your heart to ache, your tears to sting, your physical suffering to feel like it's overtaking your life. Hold onto that promise, that treasure, the new, perfected art-and-crafted masterpiece in a glorious body.

The Artist and Sculptor Himself is awaiting you in Heaven, ready to give you your new body, one free of day-in and day-out groanings and sobs; free of tubes hooked up to IVs; free of medicine that supposedly should slow your disease's progression; free from others' glares and stares; free of aches that can sometimes feel like they're suffocating your soul; free of needles, which are actually the easy part, as well as blood transfusions; free of endless nights in a cold hospital bed; free of tears staining your pillows; free of wheel chairs and surgeries, artificial limbs, and scans and X-rays; free of questions from people who don't believe you or don't understand.

You will no longer have a body that won't let you get out of bed or turn a door knob. You will cast off the body that, according to doctors, is housing a terminal disease, the body that gives you a catch in your throat and swollen circles under your eyes from crying—because of the devastating effects all this has on those you love, those who must witness the havoc and life destruction of your disease.

Those of us who live through these examples will no longer be in that body, that earthly tent, and shall one day be eternal and free of disease.

"For we know that if the earthly tent which is our house is torn down, we have a building from God, a house not made with hands, eternal in the heavens."

– 2 Corinthians 5:1

So, keep trusting, keep climbing, keep letting God and Christ be your joy and strength daily. Live with disease with hope and promise in Christ. Remember, you have salvation, forgiveness, life eternal. You have the Mighty Messiah. He is your Ultimate Sacrifice who can sympathize. Christ, the Death Conqueror, is standing with you, always with you, through your disease or disability. Continue to strive to be like Him in your given trial; one day you will reach the final rung in the Ladder, and you'll never have to take another step. You'll have reached the top, radiant glory unveiled, climbing up and out of this world, your tears wiped away and the cure before your eyes, to forever life with the Healer himself and the King of Endless Days, the King of Chronic Love, praise the Lord! Come quickly, Lord Jesus, come!

Lord,

Thank you for Your Chronic Love. Thank you for those sisters who have placed their life in Christ. Thank you for salvation and for these believing sisters living with their relentless disease or disability yet continuing daily to give You praise, honor, and glory and witness to others of Your love, mercy, and grace. Give them, and those caring for them, the strength that only You can give as well as hope that resides only in the Truth and peace of knowing You as their Lord. Give each of them the desire to show the same kind of profound Love that You showed on the cross through your steadfast sacrifice and let them be that to others. May they endure this disease or disability daily, knowing one day the promise of Heaven will be theirs. And for those who've not received forgiveness through Christ, may this be the day they receive salvation and become a new creation in Christ.

Amen.

QUESTIONS:

1. What is salvation? Do you have salvation in Christ? How do you receive salvation?

   Can you earn salvation? Why not?

2. Does having a disease or disability keep you from salvation? What does Isaiah 53:4-12 teach us? Read the verse again and write down how Christ died for you.

3. Having a disease or disability can cause great physical pain. Did Christ feel physical pain?

   Did Christ feel emotional pain? How?

4. What does the Bible tell us about our diseased body or disability when we get to heaven? Write out some verses that were used in the chapter to remind you that you'll not always have a disease or disability.

5. What are some ways you let disease or disability steal your joy?

6. Who is our Anchor? Write out the verse that tells us who our Anchor is if we are a believer. How is He our Anchor?

7. Meditate on the Good News of salvation. List some ways you see our awesome God giving you daily blessings, things for which you're thankful.

   An example: I'm thankful for salvation. I'm thankful for my adoring husband and daughter. I'm thankful for the sun rising this morning, a family who loves me, friends, etc.

8. God loves you with a Chronic Love. What does that mean? Why is that special?

9. What are a few of your favorite verses about salvation? Meditate on those and study the verses in-depth to give you encouragement.

10. What are some verses in this chapter that describe what it's like to be made new as a believer? How does this give you encouragement and an eternal perspective? Memorize one of these verses to help you when you're struggling with the emotional or physical pain of a disease or disability.

11. Write out a prayer, thanking God for salvation and what the Gospel does for you in this life spiritually.

THE CHRONIC WORD

"If we cannot all FEEL alike, we can all FEED alike on the Bread of Life."
– Charles Haddon Spurgeon
Morning and Evening
Based on the English Standard Version

In the beginning was the word and the word was with God and the word was God.
– John 1:1

Dear Precious Sister,

Hopefully, you drank in the soul-satisfying truth of Chapter Two with me, the Good News of Chronic Love and Salvation. What a jaw-dropping, life-comforting realization to know that, even if our bodies are deteriorating, our souls are free if we have repented and put our faith in Christ. So, have joy and overwhelming peace, knowing that your disease or disability is temporal, and one day we will truly be rid of all the pain, suffering, anguish, injustice, tears, and sin that now try to wage war in our bodies.

Therefore, we do not lose heart, but though our outer man is decaying, yet our inner man is being renewed day by day. For momentary, light affliction is producing for us an eternal weight of glory far beyond all comparison, while we look not at the things which are

seen, but at the things which are not seen; for the things which are
seen are temporal, but the things which are not seen are eternal.
– 2 Corinthians 4:16-17

Chapter Three is all about the Holy Book, the truth-text, the Bible. The Word of God is carved, stamped, and sealed by His blood through the many authors He had pen the scriptures. The Bible is God's infallible, inherent, inspired Word, the solid rock that Peter stood on, the firm foundation of every believer. The perfect Precepts of our Lord are the same today as when they were written 1,500 years ago. The Bible has over 40 authors and contains 66 individual books. It was originally written in three languages: Hebrew, Aramaic, and Koine Greek, and is made up of two primary parts, the Old and New Testaments. Dr. Mike Fabarez, in his amazing discipleship study called *Partners 1-on-1 Discipleship*, says this: "There should be no doubts about the accuracy of the transmission of the Bible. Those who claim that the Bible has been written and rewritten and that the message of the Bible has evolved over time are speaking from ignorance. The facts are that we have a reliable, attested record of God's Word." Dr. Fabarez uses these quotes in his discipleship book to further back the truth of the Bible:

"It may be stated categorically that no archaeological discovery has ever controverted a biblical reference."
– Nelson Glueck, *Rivers in the Desert*[2]

"The excessive skepticism shown toward the Bible by important historical schools of the eighteenth and nineteenth centuries, certain phases of which still appear periodically, has

---

2 Glueck Dr. Nelson, *Rivers in the Desert*, (New York: Farrar, Strous and Cudahy, 1959), 136.

been progressively discredited. Discovery after discovery has established the accuracy of innumerable details, and has brought increased recognition to the value of the Bible as a source of history."

– William F. Albright, *The Archaeology of Palestine*

ANCIENT WORDS

The Bible's ancient words were scribed for our salvation, protection, and growth—for our eternal hope! —to teach, sanctify, correct, and convict us, and to help us live in righteousness as a slave to Christ. The Bible is the Gospel. God selected men whom He had write the Bible, and every word is inspired and God-breathed onto the pages by the mouth of the One whom the universe magnifies. Although the Bible has different authors, all were instructed supernaturally through the Holy Spirit what to write.

"But know this first of all, that no prophecy of Scripture is a matter of one's own interpretation, for no prophecy was ever made by an act of human will, but men moved by the Holy Spirit spoke from God."

– 1 Peter 1:20-21

The Bible is the love story full of divine wonder that leads us to a wooden cross, curing sin's satisfaction. It leads us to the crass but elegant crucifixion of our Lord, who died for us to celebrate our own New Life. The Bible is God's very own words written to us, His treasured children. It's His scrolls rolled out for us in beautiful accord, telling us how to receive eternal life, with trustworthy instructions on how to live on this earth as godly women, not worldly women. The Bible is our Top Commander to fight our disease in God's army, and we must suit up in our combat gear to begin the training.

ONLY ONE WORD

Today, "the Word" means so many different, wrong things to people. It's considered no longer infallible, no longer the Truth, and can change as fast as you can unfriend someone on Facebook. For some, it's just lip service or quick assurance, a way to convince themselves they can avoid Hell. People claim to know Jesus by name and use Him an as an escape route, but they don't know Him as the Savior of the sinful who tells us we will enter only through Him, the Narrow Gate. He is not an escape route, but He is the Gate, and few will truly enter by it.

"Enter through the narrow gate; for the gate is wide and the way is broad that leads to destruction, and there are many who enter through it. For the gate is small and the way is narrow that leads to life, and there are few who find it."

– Matthew 7:13-14

For some the Bible is a way to take Truth and twist it, like trying to fit into the perfect jeans, squeezing into a size we're not, sucking in our tummies as we try to get the zipper to stay up instead of watching it slide back down and denying what the dressing room's full-length mirror is saying. Why do we want to look different than our Lord? Why is it important to wear the newest style and the latest brand—in the size we perceive that the world views as acceptance or beauty—instead of the original, genuine, and perfectly fitting garment of Christ and His Word?

WOMEN OF THE WORD, NOT THE WORLD

"The best means of resisting the devil is, to destroy whatever of the world remains in us, in order to raise for God, upon its ruins, a building all of love. Then shall we begin, in this fleeting life, to love God as we shall love him in eternity."

– John Wesley

Today for women, the Word is in grave danger of becoming extinct and no longer alive in the cannon, God's Holy pages, but morphed into words that strip women of the very essence of what we're called to be. Whether we are single or married, have a disease or not, we should live as women who love the Lord and love His Word—even though the world declares it wrong for women to have a gentle and quiet spirit, to be submissive and godly. For a wife and mother, it's no longer the norm in this culture to want to love and submit to our husband, serve our family, make dinner, go grocery shopping, clean the house, train up our children in the way of the Lord, and be above reproach in our Christian life.

> *You shall love the LORD your God with all your heart and with all your soul and with all your might. These words, which I am commanding you today, shall be on your heart. You shall teach them diligently to your sons and shall talk of them when you sit in your house and when you walk by the way and when you lie down and when you rise up.*
>
> – Deuteronomy 6:5-7

It's no longer acceptable to look and act like a Titus 2 woman:
> *Likewise, teach the older women to be reverent in the way they live, not to be slanderers or addicted to much wine, but to teach what is good. Then they can urge the younger women to love their husbands*

and children, to be self-controlled and pure, to be busy at home, to be kind, and to be subject to their husbands, so that no one will malign the word of God.

– Titus 2:3-5

Instead, so many of us are addicted to self-improvement and self-fulfillment, while Jesus taught denying self.

"Whoever does not carry his own cross and come after Me cannot be My disciple."

– Luke 14:27

THE GLASS SLIPPER FITS WHETHER YOU WEAR AN EVENING GOWN OR A HOSPITAL GOWN

Whether the carriage takes us to a ball in an elegant dress or in cotton hospital gown, God sees beauty, worth, and godliness on the inside, not in our physical looks. But still our hearts struggle; we're often frustrated in believing that being a rockstar-diva only on the outside means we have worth in the eyes of society, and we let the world's views become our drive and focus instead of God's Word and His promises:

So, as those who have been chosen of God, holy and beloved, put on a heart of compassion, kindness, humility, gentleness and patience; bearing with one another, and forgiving each other, whoever has a complaint against anyone; just as the Lord forgave you, so also should you. Beyond all these things put on love, which is the perfect bond of unity.

– Colossians 3:12

. . . not by way of eyeservice, as men-pleasers, but as slaves of Christ, doing the will of God from the heart.

– Ephesians 6:6

God's Word is golden! It gives us the mindset and Truth we vitally need through the Holy Spirit, to fend off the all-too-familiar, gross lie the fairy godmother in *Cinderella* wants us to believe: that beauty is the answer to all of life's problems. The world believes that being a "pumpkin"—a modest, godly woman concerned about the attitude of our worth in Christ—is frumpy, and instead we must be a "glass carriage," worldly and with water-downed and sometimes fake faith to fit in with a fleshly and materialistic society. Women think their cooking apron should be a sparkling, bedazzled gown that drips with diamonds, that they should look like a Disney princess, desiring outward embellishments and a fashionista's lifestyle—full of self-pride at the cost of strengthening their inward "man."

This fascination with only the "book's cover" has become our daily obsession. In discussing the development of our inward character, Andrew Murray says, "Pride needs to die in us for anything of Heaven to live in us." Some people see those with a disease or disability as different, tainted, not fully alive, not completely human. Disease or disability can scrape up our face, body, and appearance like a child scratching at a mosquito bite; and while we can't control how others see us, when we score ourselves that way, it indicates our pride at work and goes against all Christ is teaching us.

At times, we as women are judged by how well our outfit matches our necklace and if our shoes fit in with this year's top picks in *Glamour* magazine. But for us who are sick, we stay in the same comfortable, practical clothes. We live in a hospital gown or a nightgown; some of us are severely handicapped; some of us have neurological disorders; some have children paralyzed and see life moment by moment; so, of course, we won't make the best dressed list or be featured in the latest Instagram of dolled-up prima donnas. Some women with disease or disability spend days and nights at a time in bed. We don't sport boutique shirts and skinny jeans. I'm not saying that fashion is wrong but am stressing an important truth: when how we look becomes our idol, then our sin nature will dominate and not the teachings of the Life-giving Word.

This quote speaks to me, from one of America's most revered evangelists:

"The Bible will keep you from sin, or sin will keep you from the Bible."
– D.L. Moody

Christ does not look at our shiny, new bling hanging down from our neck, and He does not He care if we're able to buy the draped new tunic that all the celebrities are wearing. Our desires can become so cold when they're focused only on our self.

"Do nothing from selfishness or empty conceit, but with humility of mind regard one another as more important than yourselves."
– Philippians 2:3

And sadly, we become consumed with our material possessions as well, not what the Word says.

"For all that is in the world, the lust of the flesh and the lust of the eyes and the boastful pride of life, is not from the Father, but is from the world."
– 1 John 2:16

We must not look to the world, but to the Word. If there were a spiritual fashion show and we were modeling Christ, then we should be the first one standing in line ready to strut the Christian catwalk, ready to rock it down the spiritual runway as a model of what a woman who cherishes the Word looks like. Sisters, your disease or disability does not make you a social leper to those looking at you as Christ directs. If we are following the Good Book and what it teaches, then being made in the likeness of our Savior means that He made us each in resplendent form. Each of you is astonishing in His eyes and in those on earth who see with the eyes of Christ. We need to find our worth in Him, in His teachings and commands, not from the world's approval.

SOCIAL MEDIA ADVANCES, BUT GOD'S WORD REMAINS THE SAME

Young girls are being taught that their mother's life was stifled by the God of the Ages, by the God who never changes yet who suddenly has changed. They're being taught that the Bible is now old, out of date, and that we need new revelation to fulfill our new Wonder Woman potential. These same young women are often snipping and cutting out exactly which Scripture they want to be their next tweet, not knowing that they've completely taken the verse out of context.

For some women, it seems, our best friend is our Facebook page or Pinterest site, where we determine our sense of style and worth based on number of pin likes; this world is all about us. Social media has taken the place of morning devotions and spending time in the Bible. As such, we've become entitled women who've let outward adornment and worldly accomplishments be fashioned into a trending idol for others to take notice. We build up our egos like a closet shelf stacked with high heels, built on how many followers or hearts and smiley faces we've gleaned beside our latest post, taking credit for our accomplished goals and merits instead of honoring, thanking, and giving glory to Christ. Today, so many women have concocted a Facebook decoupage of what we want people to see, living off dreams instead of pursuing and living out the treasured reality of becoming and being a godly woman. Many Christian women are forgetting the role that God has called us to be and outlined for us in Scripture.

> *Your adornment must not be merely external—braiding the hair, and wearing gold jewelry, or putting on dresses; but let it be the hidden person of the heart, with the imperishable quality of a gentle and quiet spirit, which is precious in the sight of God. For in this way in former times the holy women also, who hoped in God, used to adorn themselves, being submissive to their own husbands.*
>
> – 1 Peter 3:3-5

The Word doesn't change. It makes us women of faith, not women of fame; it teaches us joy in submission, not to be poised to take over the nation in hopes of worldly gain and reality-TV stardom. Our power lies in understanding and studying the Bible, not studying what the world is trying to teach. In fact, they are in complete opposition: the Bible offers life while the world offers death.

> *"There is a way which seems right to a man, but its end is the way of death."*
>
> – Proverbs 14:12

KEEP IT IN CONTEXT

We as women need to know that we cannot take God's Word out of context. The Bible is sufficient, all powerful and complete, never to be added to or subtracted from, and is beautifully exhaustive and prescribed just the way our God of the Ages commanded it to be. For all women, all girls, all with diseases and disabilities, all tribes and nations, every single person who lives on this planet, the Word is the Truth, and it's the only Word.

"In the beginning was the Word and the Word was with God and the Word was God. He was with God in the beginning. Through him all things were made; without him nothing was made that has been made. In him was life and that life was the light of all mankind."

– John 1:1-4

Having a disease or disability, we should be ever mindful of flooding our hearts with Truth. We should hide God's Word in our hearts.

"How can a young man keep his way pure? By keeping it according to Your word. With all my heart I have sought You; do not let me wander from Your commandments. Your word I have treasured in my heart, that I may not sin against You."

– Psalm 119:9-11

God's Word keeps us from wanting to sin and becoming tempted to doubt, from becoming depressed and feeling hopeless with our disease. It will ring true in our hearts, clang like the brass symbols, resound and pound in our chests, and we will respond to it! We need the Word so that over and over we can hear it, memorize it, recall it to memory, and put in into practice each day.

"This book of the law shall not depart from your mouth, but you shall meditate on it day and night, so that you may be careful to do according to all that is written in it; for then you will make your way prosperous, and then you will have success."

– Joshua 1:8

The only Word that will keep us raising the battle cry of Faith and the armor of His Truth is the Bible. The Word is never to be thumbed through and skimmed over like a cultural comic book of today's Christianity. We need the Word to be able to keep our minds centered and take our thoughts captive to Christ.

> *"We are destroying speculations and every lofty thing raised up against the knowledge of God, and we are taking every thought captive to the obedience of Christ."*
>
> – 2 Corinthians 10:5

God's Word helps us recognize when we are going into the deathly war-zone against our own flesh and the enemy's ploys and tactics; and he doesn't fight fair. The enemy is there to kill and destroy.

> *"The thief comes only to steal and kill and destroy; I came that they may have life, and have it abundantly."*
>
> – John 10:10

FEMININE NOT FEMINIST

My friends and sisters, the untrue word promotes a feminist woman: a woman over her own body.

> *Therefore, I urge you, brethren, by the mercies of God, to present your bodies a living and holy sacrifice, acceptable to God, which is your spiritual service of worship. And do not be conformed to this world, but be transformed by the renewing of your mind, so that you may prove what the will of God is, that which is good and acceptable and perfect."*
>
> – Romans 12:1-2

This untrue word tells the feminist woman she's got all autonomy as her own person, a woman who controls her future and destiny, no longer needing the Scripture but what she can make it mean alongside her selfish goals and dreams.

"Do you not know that you are a temple of God and that the Spirit of God dwells in you?"
– 1 Corinthians 3:16

May the ancient text drown out those fickle, frivolous voices that have so misused God's Word. We must hold the Bible up high, and whether or not we have disease or disability, we must coil our girly fingers around it and be feminine, not a feminist. The Word is Christ! The Scripture transforms us back into women of the true Word, who find great reward in seeking to be a safe-haven of godliness and beauty on the inside, as jewels far above life's suffering, as women who fear the Lord.

Being women and young women with a daily ailment, we can still do so many things that have a spiritual impact for Christ. We can find great love in serving the Body of Christ in whatever way we can, such as devotedly praying for our pastors and others in our church body. By being an example of devotion in prayer, reading and applying God's Word, and exhibiting the fruit of the Spirit, we can be servant beacons honed on seeing the lost raised to the heights of salvation.

"But the fruit of the Spirit is love, joy, peace, patience, kindness, goodness, faithfulness, gentleness, self-control; against such things there is no law."
– Galatians 5:22-23

We should want to be like women with a servant's heart, taking a glass bowl of spiritual fruit salad to a Sunday potluck. We should be living out the God-breathed Word because we're in awesome awe and want to worship Him. We are women who won't let our disease, disability, or trials and circumstances hurt our spiritual progress and cause sin habits to form. We should not let our physical disease or disability stifle our passion or conceal our zeal for the Almighty.

We can never lose Christ, nor can we change who we are in Christ. Praise the Lord! We are forever a New Creation, but we can undermine and grow complacent and even distant to letting His Word dwell richly in us if we're listening to counsel that's not biblical, if we're not reading, studying, or listening to His Word being taught, if we're not praying to be continually sanctified, and if we're holding onto a sin pattern and not being repentant.

Are we strong warriors of the Word? Do we rely on His Truth, on His grace, love, mercy, and hope in His teachings to give us the boost we need to keep fighting disease and keep on living with joy? Feminist women who love everything of the world are living for the cheers of man. Women who are submissive because it's the call of His Word should not look or live like the world. The feminist culture and movement hate us because they feel we're a disgrace to *all* women; the world views us as meek mice with no voice, ruled by men. Feminism sees submissiveness and godliness as doormats to wipe their feet on, but this is in complete opposition to what God tells us in His Word and the kind of woman He praises.

> *"Charm is deceitful and beauty is vain, but a woman who fears the Lord, she shall be praised."*
>
> – Proverbs 31:30

One of my favorite authors says this:

"The fact that I am a woman does not make me a different kind of Christian, but the fact that I am a Christian makes me a different kind of woman."

– Elisabeth Elliot

GODLY EXAMPLE

We as Christian women are called to embrace and exhibit the characteristics of a righteous, noble woman—the virtues of a woman of faith and character—whether we're single or married, in the prime of our twenties or with laugh lines and silver hair, with or without a disease. No matter our degree of pain and suffering, we can live a purposeful life with disease or disability. Having a disease does not change Scripture or the picture of a woman's godliness; in fact, the Bible highlights and emphasizes this stunning picture. As women with disease, we love God; and just as we should as a believer, we still proclaim His love and want to live like Him. As women with disease or disability, or as caregivers of someone with a disease, we're still called to emulate and be godly women.

We are called to exhibit the bravery of Rahab, a woman who risked her life to help hide the spies when Joshua was sent out to scout out Jericho.

"When we heard it, our hearts melted and no courage remained in any man any longer because of you; for the LORD your God, He is God in heaven above and on earth beneath."

– Joshua 2:11

When the townspeople heard about God's victories, how He struck down towns like a mallet striking a bass drum, their hearts melted within them, but not so with Rahab. She recognized Him as the "Lord your God . . . God of Heaven above and on earth beneath." This harlot became a woman who, in Hebrews 11:31, is recognized in the "hall of faith." The Lord made a prostitute part of His sacred "family tree," part of the genealogy of Jesus Christ. Fourteen generations of ordinary, chosen people are part of Christ's genealogy, and the brave, cleansed, no-longer-a-prostitute Rahab is one of them.

That is the God to whom we lift our praise and worship. He took a pagan prostitute, made her a hero, saved her, and gave her access to His supernatural bloodline. Ladies, *we* cannot escape disease, but we can be courageous and fight this disease with a determined heart, brave through it all as Rahab was when she hid the men, knowing it could cost her life. We are also His daughters, and one day we will meet the saints referenced in Hebrews, and we will be like them and have a perfected faith as they do.

We should exhibit the patience, persistence, and prayer of Hannah, who sought God for a child as she waited and trusted in Him. Then Hannah, in selflessness of love, gave her child, Samuel, back to God! (1 Samuel 1:10-11). We should display the worship of Mary as she sat at Christ's feet, mesmerized by His teachings. With the same boldness for Christ, we should also display the hospitality of Lydia (Acts 16:13-15). Lydia publicly confessed Christ, was baptized, and then won her servants over for Christ as well. She showed kindness and a servant's heart by opening her home through hospitable means to Paul and Silas, after their release from prison. We should show the unconditional, sacrificial love of Moses' mother Jochebed, as she left him in the reeds of the river in a woven basket, keeping him from being killed, until he was discovered by Pharaoh's daughter. Moses' mother had to watch another woman raise Moses as her own. Can you imagine having to give your child to someone else to raise, to someone who did not believe in Christ and served other gods? (Exodus 2:1-10). We should be loyal like Esther, who showed loyalty to God and her people by standing up to the king, going boldly before him to ask for a new decree (Esther 7:1-6).

Like Rahab, Hannah, Mary, Lydia, Jochebed, and Esther—all precious, biblically empowered women—we, too, can emulate Christ as they did, showing bravery, patience, persistence in prayer, trust in God, and selflessness in love for others. We should be faithful in worship; bold in our faith and sharing the Gospel; hospitable to others; and loyal to our God—loyal, knowing He is good; loyal, continually trusting Him, knowing He purposed us and is allowing our grievance and hindering heartache to bring a greater good.

These women of the Bible held up the Truth of the Word. They displayed the character traits of Christ in their lives, and they are the examples we should replicate. We should ask God to give us the will and desire to develop the character traits of the women of ancient past to help us keep our disease from overtaking our lives in all areas. Instead of being angry and bitter about our disease, we can read the accounts of these godly women and seek God to strengthen our hearts, character, minds, and spiritual life as He did theirs. The accounts of these women point to their spiritual accomplishments because they ultimately had faith, a solid trust in God and what the Bible teaches. These accounts are not recorded for us to learn we need big girly muscles or a healthy physical body. These women may have been physically strong on the outside, but more importantly, we need to know how they looked on the inside. We know they had a deep reverence for the Lord. The spotlight is on their character; they illustrate what we should be like as well.

Former First Lady Eleanor Roosevelt said this:

"A woman is like a tea bag;
you never know how strong it is until it's in hot water."

The very nature of being a woman who follows Christ is one who follows His teachings, spending time reading the Bible and serving the living God. Being sick cannot keep us from worshiping our God. We worship God in Spirit and in Truth.

"God is spirit, and those who worship Him must worship in spirit
and truth."

– John 4:24

The truth is . . . worship is not just singing and praising Him through song; we also worship in Truth by following and believing what the Word teaches; the Bible is the Truth. Worship is giving God esteem and honor, grateful for each moment on this earth, even with our weary and tired bodies because we celebrate that we won't always be sick. Salvation guarantees us spiritual health. When we are received into Heaven, our health will be 100% perfect. We will have no more sorrow and no more death; no plaguing disease or terminal prognosis; no congenital birth defects or paralysis; no more trying to fix a broken body or change deformed cells.

KNOW THE WORD

As a woman having a disease, life is exhausting. And so many times, we just want to quit fighting; we want to throw in the towel. But if we know the Word and put the verses into practice, we can fight and will receive the crown at the end of earthly life. You must know that on those days, when our spiritual nourishment of contentment, joy, trust, and faith is lacking, we need to bulk up on the meat and bread of His Word, feed our starved soul, and then sit back on a full stomach and be satisfied in the Truth:

> *But He answered and said, "It is written, 'Man shall not live on bread alone, but on every word that proceeds out of the mouth of God'."*
>
> – Matthew 4:4

We are powerless and vulnerable to the world's fad teachings if we do not understand the Word of God. We could get sucked in by teachings that claim it's our fault we have a disease, that we obviously aren't filled with the Spirit and simply need to claim our healing in "faith." Wrong counsel allows you to demand your own way with God. It influences tell you to "use this essential oil," "do this work-out routine," "try this diet," "pray this prayer," "go see this holistic doctor," "pay this money to receive a healing vile of medicine," or "use this handkerchief prayed over by a faith healer."

You name it, they're selling it. We don't need to try and overcome our disease or disability with these promised quick fixes. Some vitamins and supplements are not bad and are healthy for the body. We also have good doctors and medicine, but if they become our heart's only desire, our idol, the place we're putting our hope and trust instead of in God and His will, we are sinning. Whether His will is for physical healing or for you to have a terminal illness and only six more months on earth, the living God is good, and your soul is alive. Your body may give way, but He promises something even better—and it, my sweet friend, will last forever. We will see His glory, His forever presence as we stand in the light, the Son of His Glory and Radiance. Hang on! He promised physical healing in Heaven, but on earth we will have troubles and suffering because He suffered, too.

> *"For just as the sufferings of Christ are ours in abundance, so also our comfort is abundant through Christ."*
> – 2 Corinthians 1:5

STRENGTHENED BY THE WORD

> *"Heaven and Earth will pass away, but my words will not pass away."*
> – Matthew 24:35

All throughout the Bible, we see people healed physically but not spiritually. We see Christ Himself walk through villages and heal people, knowing full well that was their only desire; they wanted Christ, not for salvation but to save them from physical pain. But we certainly see the opposite as well. We see people who are beaten, with their cities desolated, who are sanctified in the Word as followers of Christ, yet who suffer intense persecution. We see all the disciples die as martyrs (except John, who was left to die on Patmos), and still through it all, they are praising, singing, and counting it worthy to have their life taken in horrific, torturous ways for the glory of seeing Him again one day. They know they'll again see the God-man, with whom they set sail, with whom they shared communion, the One they cherished not only as their Lord and Master but as their Brother as outcasts in society.

The churches, the saints, are giving Him glory, even when they're wailing in lament over their church buildings in rubble; even when they're on the run, scattered, hiding as hunted sojourners, and threatened with death for standing with Christ, for drawing the Christian fish in the sand and identifying themselves as believers. They're standing on His Word, the source of their bravery, power, hope, and love. His Word is their strength to be counted worthy to suffer—some even seeing their pleading, screaming children ripped from their arms and dragged away to be murdered or carted off and taken as slaves. Their faith is in the Word, and they won't recant. Their faith is not in cures, diets, protein shakes, or modern culture's infomercials that promise success, power in money, and "miracle cures" that, for the right price, can raise someone from the dead.

"Yes, in just three easy payments of $29.95 plus shipping and handling, you'll receive the book by the latest breakout, false teacher and get a free scented candle to ward off evil as a bonus!"—or something similar we hear blare in our ears, like a late-night infomercial on TV. Bogus and unsettling in our soul, these pitches have nothing to do with the Sovereign Savior and have contorted the Word like a circus sideshow act.

Read the Word. He gave us the Word to give us eternal life, to help us look at life through the lens of eternity. Our physical body will plague us only right now; just like snapping your finger, it will soon be gone. Don't buy into anything other than His Word. Remember, the truths we should really be swallowing as a multi-vitamin for a fit, strong, spiritual body is the Word and its counsel.

FALSE PEDDLERS

In 2 Timothy 4, Paul is exhorting Timothy to preach the Word; he warns him about the false teachers to come, a strong warning we need to hear as well:

> I solemnly charge you in the presence of God and of Christ Jesus, who is to judge the living and the dead, and by His appearing and His kingdom: preach the word; be ready in season and out of season; reprove, rebuke, exhort, with great patience and instruction. For the time will come when they will not endure sound doctrine; but wanting to have their ears tickled, they will accumulate for themselves

*teachers in accordance to their own desire, and will turn away their
ears from the truth and will turn aside to myths. But you, be sober
in all things, endure hardship, do the work of an evangelist, fulfill
your ministry.*

– 2 Timothy 4:1-5

I know you hear things that tickle your ears, that can make you
believe you have the faith to cure yourself, or that if you would just
pray a little harder and have more faith, your disease would be healed.
This is completely and utterly false. Your disease or disability can be
healed, but only if it's God's will. Unless it's in God's Word and taught
in context, then what you are hearing preached or read in a Christian
book is being peddled falsely under the name of Christ; it's not the
Truth of the Bible but a fake, musty potion of ignorance, lies, personal
gain, and even some blasphemy thrown in. The Bible warns us that
many will come in His name.

*"But even if we, or an angel from heaven, should preach to you
a gospel contrary to what we have preached to you, he is to
be accursed!"*

– Galatians 1:8

But we know who Christ is and what He did.

We know what the Word teaches us about suffering and trials. We
know that for some of us, our suffering could take our life. Giving us
insight today, Paul wrote to Timothy and the church in Corinth about
the affliction he experienced in Asia.

*For just as the sufferings of Christ are ours in abundance, so also
our comfort is abundant through Christ. But if we are afflicted, it
is for your comfort and salvation; or if we are comforted, it is for
your comfort, which is effective in the patient enduring of the same*

sufferings which we also suffer; and our hope for you is firmly
grounded, knowing that as you are sharers of our sufferings, so also
you are sharers of our comfort.
                                        – 2 Corinthians 1:5-7

For some of us, being in the middle of a trial means our suffering persists at length or is progressing into something worse . . . but this is not the end. God was aware of His chosen people suffering in Egypt under Pharaoh's hand.

"The Lord said, 'I have surely seen the affliction of My people who are
in Egypt, and have given heed to their cry because of their taskmas-
ters, for I am aware of their sufferings'."
                                        – Exodus 3:7

God sees our sufferings, too. He sees our affliction and gives heed to our cry, just as He did for His chosen in Egypt. We are His chosen in Christ, and we are His people. You are His child, and He sees all you endure daily. He hears your personal woes and pleas when you cry out to Him. When you read His Word, you are hearing His voice through Scripture, and He will build you up, toughened and reinforced with Truth. The Truth of God's Word is our personal trainer at the gym, pushing us to pump up with "holy iron" to bolster our spiritual body. The Bible gives us the words the Lord wrote for us, inspirational words transcribed through chosen men; these men he chose to indwell with the Holy Spirit, so they could compose each word, verse, chapter, and book, including the Truth of how to live with disease or disability. The Truth for our lives is found through the Word, and that's all we need.

LIVING LIKE A WARRIOR

God's Word holds the key that unlocks the facts we need to fight the enemy, to be godly women who can ward off our assailant. We have three enemies: Satan, our flesh, and . . . the Fall. If we live with our disease as our idol, trying to beat it, understand it, or deny it, living in our flesh like the "old man" we once were, we will lose not only the first battle and every battle thereafter, but ultimately, we will succumb to letting our disease win the war.

> "... that, in reference to your former manner of life, you lay aside
> the old self, which is being corrupted in accordance with the lusts of
> deceit, and that you be renewed in the spirit of your mind, and put
> on the new self, which in the likeness of God has been created in
> righteousness and holiness of the truth."
>
> – Ephesians 4:22-24

God's Word gives us hope and security that this disease is not forever; His Word holds every answer we need to battle our enemy and keep our minds and thoughts on heavenly things, upward realities. The Word teaches us how to see, view, and live with our disease. The Bible teaches us that in our former life, before we were Christians, we were being darkened in our understanding.

> "... being darkened in their understanding, excluded from the life of
> God because of the ignorance that is in them, because of the hard-
> ness of their heart."
>
> – Ephesians 4:18

Once we are a Christian, no longer in the dark but having the light of Scripture, we understand that our disease should not dictate our day-to-day life—as well as our ultimate destiny—and how it makes us feel about ourselves, others, and God Himself. It should not cause us to sin against our God or others in our thoughts, motives, and actions. The Bible gives us the spiritual enablement to fight by the very words of Scripture.

JOY COMES IN THE MORNING

Friend, when I wake up, I want my day to begin with me knowing I'm joyful with this disease. Joyful doesn't mean I'm excited I have a disease but that I can find contentment in my circumstances. When I wake, I'm confident I can defeat my foe head to head—the foe of my flesh, the foe of Satan, and the world's views—in one-on-one combat, and that I won't let my disease steal my joy. Our Mighty Warrior teaches us through His Word to fight the good fight, and when we think we're failing, to keep fighting and know that the battle is lifelong, that it takes great patience and is not for the faint of heart. And that's when we must put on our spiritual armor and slay the dragon. We are knights in shining armor, the blazing armor of our Lord. We must put on the full armor of God; we must battle every day:

> *Finally, be strong in the Lord and in the strength of His might. Put on the full armor of God, so that you will be able to stand firm against the schemes of the devil. For our struggle is not against flesh and blood, but against the rulers, against the powers, against the world forces of this darkness, against the spiritual forces of wickedness in the heavenly places. Therefore, take up the full armor of God, so that you will be able to resist in the evil day, and having done everything, to stand firm. Stand firm therefore, having girded your loins with truth, and having put on the breastplate of righteousness, and having shod your feet with the preparation of the gospel of peace; in addition to all, taking up the shield of faith with which you will be able to extinguish all the flaming arrows of the evil one. And take the helmet of salvation, and the sword of the Spirit, which is the word of God. With all prayer and petition pray at all times in the Spirit, and with this*

*in view, be on the alert with all perseverance and petition for all
the saints.*

– Ephesians 6:10-18

CHRIST, THE PHYSICAL WORD

The Word is referring to Christ Himself. He is the Bread of Life,
the perfected in bone. Jesus, the Word, is Chronic. We have the ability
through His Word to be sustained. Before everything—time, space, matter, chasms of continuum, the cosmos, and the earth—was the Word.

*"In the beginning was the Word, and the Word was with God, and the
Word was God."*

– John 1:1

Before disease, sin, and death, there was the Word. Jesus was there
when God and the Holy Spirit created the earth and the heavens and
set into motion His plan for your individual life.

*"In the beginning God created the heavens and the earth. The earth
was formless and void, and darkness was over the surface of the deep,
and the Spirit of God was moving over the surface of the waters."*

– Genesis 1:1-2

*Then God said, "Let Us make man in Our image, according to Our
likeness; and let them rule over the fish of the sea and over the birds
of the sky and over the cattle and over all the earth, and over every
creeping thing that creeps on the earth." God created man in His
own image, in the image of God He created him; male and female
He created them. God blessed them; and God said to them, "Be
fruitful and multiply, and fill the earth, and subdue it; and rule*

over the fish of the sea and over the birds of the sky and over every
living thing that moves on the earth."
                                    – Genesis 1:26-28

God spoke the Word and creation began. God gave us the Word in the flesh, who is His Son, Jesus Christ.

"But as many as received Him, to them He gave the right to be-
come children of God, even to those who believe in His name, who
were born, not of blood nor of the will of the flesh nor of the will of
man, but of God. And the Word became flesh, and dwelt among us,
and we saw His glory, glory as of the only begotten from the Father,
full of grace and truth."
                                    – John 1:12-14

He purposed for the Word to be born of a virgin by the Holy Spirit, grow as a child, become a man with an ultimate, non-negotiable plan, die on the cross, take on our sin, and be raised from the dead. He is a Person, the second in the Trinity. The Word is a man; the Word is the Son of God; and the Word is Christ.

"And the Word became flesh, and dwelt among us, and we saw His
glory, glory as of the only begotten from the Father, full of grace
and truth."
                                    – John 1:14

I cannot say that enough to myself and to you. When you feel like you are lost, not able to find your way out, when you find yourself back in the dark pit, your hands aching from climbing the ladder, hold on, re-grip the rungs, and remember Christ is a person. He was a person, just like you and me.

For His thirty-three years on earth, He lived as a nomad, not the conqueror of nations the Jews hoped for, but He was the conqueror of sin. He was tortured and gave His life for us. He really existed, and He really was crucified for you and me as believers. He felt pain, He laughed, He loved, He lived. He grew up as a little boy with brothers and sisters, and He had a job as a carpenter. He was poor, a nobody in what was important. But He was born with a King's blood, blood that left His body when His life was taken from Him as a man, but also as our God. Our God, Our Christ, is our Word as well as our saving God-man.

Every emotion you have felt with your disease, Jesus has felt, too, but the difference is this: since He was perfect, He did not sin in His emotions. As believers, we must make that truth an "aha moment" in our minds forever; we must stamp it with a permanent tattoo on our hearts, and we must brand it in our minds like a cowboy making it clear just which cattle are his. We are branded by the Truth of the Word in our hearts, and it will never be removed. When people see you, they should see Christ working in you.

"God who foresaw your tribulation has specially armed you to go through it, Not without pain but without stain."

– C.S. Lewis

CHRIST, THE WRITTEN WORD

Christ is not only the physical Word Himself; He is the Divine Inspiration written on the pages of the Bible, the Holy written Word. Teaching on the self-expression of God, which is the Truth of His Word, John MacArthur states, "Of course, there cannot be any discord or difference of opinion between the *written* Word of God (Scripture) and the *incarnate* Word of God (Jesus). In the first place, truth cannot contradict itself. Second, Scripture is called 'the word of Christ' (Colossians 3:16). It is *His* message, *His* self-expression. In other words, the Truth of Christ and the Truth of the Bible are of the very same character. They are in perfect agreement in every respect. Both are equally true. God has revealed Himself to humanity through Scripture and through His Son. Both perfectly embody the essence of what truth is."[3]

Our disease has a purpose, and the God of endless days will use it and perfect us through it if we live lives set apart for Him. We do not have to be the kid being bullied; we can walk into school with the Word at our side, protecting us from the bully's blows. Although we have a defining disease, when we pray, we're talking to the One who made matter, space, and the continuum of time, and who made you, my friend. He will give you immovable strength with this disease or disability to use the Word rightly—to receive the spiritual vigor and direction you need to uphold His commands and adhere to His encouraging counsel.

A HEART FOR GOD'S WORD

Christ as our Word offers us salvation, regeneration and sanctification, repentance, faith, deliverance from sin, and entrance to blissful eternity, just to name a few. The Bible is alive because Christ and the words He spoke are living through Scripture. The Word is living and active, sharper than any two-edged sword.

> *"For the word of God is living and active and sharper than any two-edged sword, and piercing as far as the division of soul and spirit, of both joints and marrow, and able to judge the thoughts and intentions of the heart."*
> – Hebrews 4:12

Christ knows our motives, our planned deeds, before we even act on them. He knows our every thought before we even speak it. He

---

3 MacArthur, John. *The Truth War: Fighting for Certainty in an Age of Deception.* Nashville: Thomas Nelson, 2008, 3.

knows our struggles, and He lets us know that we are responsible for the actions and intents of our heart:

> *O Lord, You have searched me and known me.*
> *You know when I sit down and when I rise up;*
> *You understand my thought from afar.*
> *You scrutinize my path and my lying down,*
> *And are intimately acquainted with all my ways.*
> *Even before there is a word on my tongue,*
> *Behold, O Lord, You know it all.*
> *You have enclosed me behind and before,*
> *And laid Your hand upon me.*
> *Such knowledge is too wonderful for me;*
> *It is too high, I cannot attain to it.*
>
> – Psalm 139:1-6

We are to keep our hearts clean, our thoughts and deeds pure, thinking only on true things while battling disease and not giving in to the negative ways it can cause us to sin.

> *"The heart is more deceitful than all else and is desperately sick;*
> *Who can understand it? I, the Lord, search the heart, I test the mind,*
> *even to give to each man according to his ways, according to the*
> *results of his deeds."*
>
> – Jeremiah 17:9-10

Our hearts give ourselves away and reveal if we truly trust Him or not. Do you truly desire His will, His plan, and are you willing to be filled with exuberant joy through this trial? Our hearts are still responsible for our actions, thoughts, and words. With our bodies sick or well, our hearts should desire Christ and look like Him.

> *"As in water face reflects face, so the heart of man reflects man."*
>
> – Proverbs 27:19

"Create in me a clean heart, O God, and renew a steadfast spirit within me."

–Psalm 51:10

THE HELPER

When we become new creations in Christ, the Holy Spirit comes to live within us.

"When the Helper comes, whom I will send to you from the Father, that is the Spirit of truth who proceeds from the Father, He will testify about Me, and you will testify also, because you have been with me from the beginning."

– John 15:26-27

The Holy Spirit is God, the third in the Trinity. The Trinity is God in three Persons, which is the God the Father, God the Son, and God the Holy Spirit.

"The grace of the Lord Jesus Christ, and the love of God, and the fellowship of the Holy Spirit, be with you all."

– 2 Corinthians 13:14

When Jesus appeared to the disciples to tell them He was leaving and going to prepare a place for them, He also left them the Holy Spirit.

"I will ask the Father, and He will give you another Helper, that He may be with you forever; that is the Spirit of truth, whom the world cannot receive, because it does not see Him or know Him, but you know Him because He abides with you and will be in you."

– John 14:16-17

Jesus left the disciples with the Helper.

"These things I have spoken to you while abiding with you. But the Helper, the Holy Spirit, whom the Father will send in My

name, He will teach you all things, and bring to your remembrance
all that I said to you."
　　　　　　　　　　　　　　　　　　　　　– John 14:25-26

As a Christian when you receive salvation, you are born-again, not of flesh, but of the Holy Spirit who now dwells inside you.

"That which is born of the flesh is flesh, and that which is born of the
Spirit is spirit. Do not be amazed that I said to you, 'You must be
born again.' The wind blows where it wishes and you hear the sound
of it, but do not know where it comes from and where it is going; so
is everyone who is born of the Spirit."
　　　　　　　　　　　　　　　　　　　　　– John 3:6-8

We have the same Holy Spirit living within us as did the disciples, who were commissioned to take the Gospel and the love of Jesus to the world. As believers, we are called and mandated to obey the Word, to live by it, and proclaim it to others. Christ also gives us a supernatural relationship to the counselor, the Holy Spirit.

"Now He who establishes us with you in Christ and anointed us is
God, who also sealed us and gave the Spirit in our hearts as a pledge."
　　　　　　　　　　　　　　　　　　　　　– 2 Corinthians 1:21-22

THE HOLY SPIRIT

Remember, the Holy Spirit makes it possible to look like Christ. He is the One who gives us conviction; He changes us from the inside:

But when the kindness of God our Savior and His love for mankind
appeared, He saved us, not on the basis of deeds which we have done
in righteousness, but according to His mercy, by the washing of regen-
eration and renewing by the Holy Spirit, whom He poured out upon

us richly through Jesus Christ our Savior, so that being justified by His
grace we would be made heirs according to the hope of eternal life.
– Titus 3:4-7

Why do we have the Holy Spirit? One reason is so when we read the Word, we can understand it. He will conform us to the image of Christ, making us grow up in our faith by transforming our minds through the text.

"And do not be conformed to this world, but be transformed by the re-
newing of your mind, so that you may prove what the will of God is,
that which is good and acceptable and perfect."
– Romans 12:2

Sisters, when your mind is consumed with the Truth and you're letting His Word thrive in your heart, then your actions will follow. With disease, the Word keeps us from anger, depression, sin, doubt, fear, and anxiety as so many verses speak directly to our minds, giving us the tools to use as our dagger of veracity, thrusting and puncturing the wicked one.

For though we walk in the flesh, we do not war according to the
flesh, for the weapons of our warfare are not of the flesh, but di-
vinely powerful for the destruction of fortresses. We are destroying
speculations and every lofty thing raised up against the knowledge
of God, and we are taking every thought captive to the obedience
of Christ."
– 2 Corinthians 10:3-5

The Holy Spirit is our soul's Best Friend, our Spiritual Comforter, and our Supreme Counselor. When we read and take in Scripture, He gives us the ability to be changed by it.

"He saved us, not on the basis of deeds which we have done in righteousness, but according to His mercy, by the washing of regeneration and renewing by the Holy Spirit."

– Titus 3:5

We become wiser and braver, strengthened by Scripture, and able to put off our flesh. We can fight the wrong thoughts and doubts that rise in our hearts due to disease or disability, and instead, trust in the Bible.

". . . that, in reference to your former manner of life, you lay aside the old self, which is being corrupted in accordance with the lusts of deceit, and that you be renewed in the spirit of your mind, and put on the new self, which in the likeness of God has been created in righteousness and holiness of the truth."

– Ephesians 4:22-24

As women with disease or disability or as caregivers, the Holy Spirit is what we need to survive our trials. God changes us through His Spirit.

WHAT DO I PRAY?

When we don't know what to do or what to pray because our disease causes us great turmoil—the aches and pains making us feel like pulverized, hammered pieces of raw meat, flattened beyond recognition, our body aching more than we thought physically possible, and we're hurting so much that words of prayer cannot come—we have the Spirit to help us pray.

"In the same way the Spirit also helps our weakness; for we do not know how to pray as we should, but the Spirit Himself intercedes for us with groanings too deep for words; and He who searches the

hearts knows what the mind of the Spirit is, because He intercedes
for the saints according to the will of God."
– Romans 8:26-27

My strong friend, the Holy Spirit is ready to give you the words to pray when you're walking down the cold hospital corridor, your dangling IV attached and barely able to keep your decrepit frame from hitting the floor after finishing another chemo treatment, and the doctor, walking slowly and eyeing his clipboard, tells you the fateful news, his words burrowing a hole in your soul like a frantic mole clawing his way underground to avoid the sun.

My sister, the Holy Spirit is ready to comfort you, giving you words to pray when you get a phone call confirming the diagnosis, the sound of your rapidly beating heart piercing your ears as the news sinks in that a certain, insidious disease will be attempting to steal your body and chop it up like a knife dicing an onion—or when your husband goes to the doctor because he has started slurring his words and is diagnosed with ALS.

My fellow suffering soul on this Chronic journey, the Holy Spirit knows your pain and is ready to help you pray when your son is born and the tests prove the unacceptable, with the survival rate only five percent; or when you beg the Lord to give you the disease, instead of helplessly watching your child hurting with disease every moment of every day of his or her life—other children growing strong and healthy while your child is happy to just be able to get outside in the wheelchair for some fresh air.

The Holy Spirit is ready to help, comfort, and sustain you when you're struck with a disease or disability that you feel strips you of your right to be an effective mom and wife, scared of the future, as the disease keeps you from participating in life events with your husband, children, church friends, and family.

Remember, we have the Spirit inside us. We have Him, and He expresses His love for us to God the Father through the prayers He prays for us. Yes, we can be assured the Holy Spirit is ready to pray, to present our needs to Jesus, who will intercede, to offer His hand and communicate with our Supreme Father. And in that hope comes the Truth that Christ is there to co-pilot the plane and get your prayers to Heaven. We know this through His Word, describing how Christ sits at the Father's right hand, interceding for us.

> *". . . who is the one who condemns? Christ Jesus is He who died, yes, rather who was raised, who is at the right hand of God, who also intercedes for us."*
>
> – Romans 8:34

Our superior and always caring God gives us the Spirit to pray for us when we just don't have the words. When your words couldn't possibly express or convey what needs said in prayer, your heart unable to express the thoughts in your mind, the Spirit knows exactly what to say and does it for you. Awake, asleep, whether you're happy or feel like you've been whittled down to tiny splinters of kindling with no spark to start a fire, like a campfire dying down in the wee hours of the cool night—no matter what you feel pain-wise, physical or emotional—nothing keeps Him from praying for what you need. Your disease has no bearing on our perfect Spirit communicating with the Son as He intercedes on your behalf to the Father. Your prayers are always heard because of the Spirit always praying. He is always praying for you:

. . . who is the one who condemns? Christ Jesus is He who died, yes, rather who was raised, who is at the right hand of God, who also intercedes for us. Who will separate us from the love of Christ? Will tribulation, or distress, or persecution, or famine, or nakedness, or peril, or sword? Just as it is written, "For your sake we are being put to death all day long; we were considered as sheep to be slaughtered." But in all these things we overwhelmingly conquer through Him who loved us."

– Romans 8:34-37

WE ARE MORE THAN CONQUERORS WITH THE WORD!

John MacArthur says this about who the Spirit is and His role in a believer's life:

"Let me tell you something: you must get this, that the Spirit's ministry in you, the Spirit's teaching ministry, the anointing in you, is to teach you the meaning of the Bible, the meaning of Scripture. It's not about esoteric extrabiblical inspiration, or some revelation out of the air; the Spirit's anointing ministry teaches you all things, and the all things that He teaches you are the all things that He has revealed in the Scripture. He is the interpreter of Scripture to the faithful student. This is His ministry."[4]

I don't think we as women realize how wise, brave, discerning, loved, empowered, and gifted we are because of the Spirit. If we as Christians could understand what the Spirit can do in our lives, we would be able to withstand the trials of disease or disability without fear, without being susceptible to our weak carnality, and our sneaky tempter; we would be able to face it with more confidence,

4 "The Illuminating Role of the Holy Spirit." Grace to You, May 3, 2015. https://www.gty.org/library/sermons-library/43-76/the-illuminating-role-of-the-holy-spirit.

knowing He is working in us to make us look like Christ. He is the One who lives within us and who gives us the eyes and ears to see, hear, and understand the Word. And we have the ability through the Holy Spirit working in us to give God praise and rejoice. It will never be easy, but it will always be possible if we live by His Word. Study it, keep it in context, memorize it, apply it. May you be new, not old.

> *"For whatever was written in earlier times was written for our in-struction, so that through perseverance and the encouragement of the Scriptures we might have hope."*
> – Romans 15:4

PRAYING THE WORD

Prayer should always be about wanting God's will, and it's always about God's glory, giving Him the highest adoration. As we go through the trials of disease or disability and the unexpected happens—like when we find out our disease or disability is terminable or incurable; or when they find a golf-ball size tumor in our child's developing body; or when your daughter is in a car wreck and suffers massive brain damage; or when your husband has a stroke and you're now the one to dress, feed, and bathe him; or when your son goes off to war and comes back without his arms because of a roadside bomb; or when you're diagnosed with Lupus, cancer, or MS; or when your child is born with congenital defects—whatever the circumstance, know God is with you through each moment. Throughout each moment of fear—whether shown in a waterfall of tears as we cower in a corner from the sad news we receive, or whether the one we love finally fades away at the hospital, leaving us to somehow face life without them—know He is with us, and He never leaves us alone.

"The Lord also will be a stronghold for the oppressed, a stronghold in times of trouble; and those who know Your name will put their trust in You, for You, O Lord, have not forsaken those who seek You."

– Psalm 9:9-10

As David tells us so beautifully, He is worthy of our praise. *"Every day I will bless You, and I will praise Your name forever and ever. Great is the Lord, and highly to be praised, and His greatness is unsearchable."*

– Psalm 145:2-3

Understanding how to pray is understanding how we should communicate with our Father, so He can hear us . . .

"I have called upon You, for You will answer me, O God; incline Your ear to me, hear my speech."

– Psalm 17:6

So He can strengthen us . . .

"My soul weeps because of grief; strengthen me according to Your word."

– Psalm 119:28

So He can comfort us . . .

"God is our refuge and strength, a very present help in trouble."

– Psalm 46:1

We need Him to change us and grow us and help us become more like His Son. We know that the words we pray are what will give us courage because they are heard. When we need strength, rest, hope, encouragement, healing . . . He hears us, and He answers. Furthermore, His answer is always to help us and for His glory to be on display.

*"For the eyes of the Lord are toward the righteous, and His ears attend
to their prayer, but the face of the Lord is against those who do evil."*
— 1 Peter 3:12

When we pray for healing, He will always do what's best for us,
but we may or may not receive healing; God has a plan, which may
not be for our healing. Our suffering may lead others to fall on the
mercy of Christ and be saved; that's why we should want God's will
to be done. The Bible confirms this:

*"Now the God of peace, who brought up from the dead the great
Shepherd of the sheep through the blood of the eternal covenant, even Jesus our Lord, equip you in every good thing to
do His will, working in us that which is pleasing in His sight,
through Jesus Christ, to whom be the glory forever and
ever. Amen."*
— Hebrews 13:20-21

So, use your megaphone to crank out your prayers, and know that
His will is always accomplished. God is listening.

TRUST IN THE WORD

He is the Word, and He has given us His Word when we hurt.
Whether we ache with disease, celebrate life, mourn, suffer loss
. . . He is our Word. He is always our Word. Though our Bible sometimes lies buried at the bottom of the bills, under junk mail on our
kitchen counters, stuffed on a shelf collecting dust, or squished in
our purse between an old piece of spearmint gum and a stretched out,
emergency hair band, it remains God's Word to you and me. It should
be our most valued, most prized, most costly possession, not just another item shoved in our purse, left on our kitchen counter, or stuffed

on a bookshelf. The Word is inspired; it is the Truth, filled with His commands, encouragement, correction, training, teaching, and rebuke.

> *"All Scripture is inspired by God and profitable for teaching, for reproof, for correction, for training in righteousness; so that the man of God may be adequate, equipped for every good work."*
>
> – 2 Timothy 3:16-17

The Bible is His heart and love, His Chronic Word poured out to us; it's the most valued, hearty, and moving gift we have in this life.

The words of Christ are inspired. The biblical definition of inspired means God- breathed. God is divine, and the writers of the Bible were supernaturally instructed what to write—His exact words. There are no errors in the Bible because it came directly from Him.

> *"But know this first, that no prophecy of Scripture is a matter of one's own interpretation, for no prophecy was ever made by an act of human will, but men moved by the Holy Spirit spoke from God."*
>
> – Peter 1:20-21

The word prophecy in this previous verse means all of Scripture. As John MacArthur said in his sermon on *Understanding the Doctrine of Inspiration,* "It means to stand before and speak *propheteia,* to speak before to disclose, to talk in front of someone, to tell forth, all that God has spoken, all that God has said, all that God has told in the Scripture."[5]

> *It's not up for debate or your interpretation. It is His book, and He is the divine author. We have the Word of Christ, and we can hear it taught and read it for ourselves. We are called to study it, sing it, pray it, meditate on it, and memorize it, to follow its teachings and commands; and*

---

5 "Understanding the Doctrine of Inspiration." Grace to You, October 29, 2006. https://www.gty.org/library/sermons-library/90-324/understanding-the-doctrine-of-inspiration.

when we do, we can simply know that when we think we can't muster
one more breath, when we become anxious and worried, then we can
pray this Truth: Be anxious for nothing, but in everything by prayer
and supplication with thanksgiving let your requests be made known
to God. And the peace of God, which surpasses all comprehension,
will guard your hearts and your minds in Christ Jesus.
– Philippians 4:6-7

He will carry you. He will wrap His invisible wings around you
and rock you, put peace over your war, sing over your fragmented
heart, and hold you up as you try to slink down and retreat. He will
supernaturally do this through the peace that passes all understanding in Christ. He gives answers to questions in such a way we just
don't understand as humans; yet this kind of help He gives protects
our heart and mind.

"I pray that the eyes of your heart may be enlightened, so that you
will know what is the hope of His calling, what are the riches of the
glory of His inheritance in the saints."
– Ephesians 1:18

The pain might still be there, but you will find His peace, courage,
and strength as you disclose your many prayers and petitions without
any fear or trepidation. Just as we imagine the lion lying with the lamb
on plush grass, at rest in the millennial kingdom, the peace of God
will quiet you, and you'll find serenity over pain, knowing you can
pray to Him, call on Him, petition Him, and cry out to Him about all
you encounter and must shoulder; you will know He is supernaturally
protecting you in Christ.

"But let all who take refuge in You be glad, let them

ever sing for joy; and may You shelter them, that those who love Your
name may exult in You."

– Psalm 5:11

We are not alone. His love calls us and propels us to keep going in our brokenness, just as Christ lifted His cup the night of the Last Supper, offering His blood and breaking bread, signifying His body being broken. As He washed even the feet of Judas, the disciple who would betray Him, and in all the many times He could have forfeited our souls to Hell, He never failed. Love never failed on the cross. He never failed us, not then and not now:

> *. . . knowing that Christ, having been raised from the dead, is never to die again; death no longer is master over Him. For the death that He died, He died to sin once for all; but the life that He lives, He lives to God. Even so consider yourselves to be dead to sin, but alive to God in Christ Jesus.*

– Romans 6:9-11

TAKE HEART

Take heart, lift your eyes, and sing praises to the Infallible, Chronic Word, the One who gives you answers to the tests of life. When you are spending days in bed, having to watch from the couch as your child leaves to go to her soccer game . . . when you have pain from joints and nerves, a sour stomach from a new pill, or another medical test looming . . . when friends turn on you and make fun of you because you look different . . . when you see your spouse struggling to cope with disease or disability and are unable to help him—when you face any of the myriad of trials that come with disease—do not let the missiles with a direct hit on your life cause you to sin. Sin is like the dragon that guards the tower, pacing in the mossy moat, breathing his sin-saturated fire at our Knight, our Savior, the charming Prince. Jesus is fulfilling the drawn-up and carried-out rescue mission of saving our hearts from this temporary, dragon-filled world. And our great Prince of Peace will return one day as a riveting King in all His splendor and majesty, commanding His army from the sky, atop a white steed, and He will destroy the slovenly effects on this earth:

> *And I saw heaven opened, and behold, a white horse, and He who sat on it is called Faithful and True, and in righteousness He judges and wages war. His eyes are a flame of fire, and on His head are many diadems; and He has a name written on Him which no one knows except Himself. He is clothed with a robe dipped in blood, and His name is called The Word of God. And the armies which are in heaven, clothed in fine linen, white and clean, were following Him on white horses. From His mouth comes a sharp sword, so that with it He may strike down the nations, and He will rule them with a rod of iron; and He treads the wine press of the fierce wrath of God, the Almighty. And on His robe and on His thigh He has a name written, "KING OF KINGS, AND LORD OF LORDS."*
>
> – Revelation 19:11-16

Sisters, remember in this life there will be famine and poverty, injustice and suffering, and we will always be fighting to cure diseases or disabilities because we live in this unclean world, but we need to keep training and dueling, swinging our sword—God's unchanging Word—to conquer the enemy, which is our flesh and Satan. If we trust in the Word and that He will deliver on His promises, our faith will stand strong as we keep contesting our disease and the impact it can make on our hearts, minds, thoughts, words, and deeds. When we are constantly bombarded by the fire-breathing dragon of sin, which is trying to keep God's Word from working in our lives, we should always fight, using that same powerful Word. We know our Knight on a white horse will come one day for all those in Christ, pull down the drawbridge, break down the door, and rescue us from sin and disease. The enemy will try to take your mind and fill it with doubt, casting a dark shroud when you're most vulnerable and losing ground, but the dark cannot hide the lit fire of His Word that makes us like irrepressible flames. Our lives, even with disease, belong to the Word, and He comforts us spiritually throughout our afflictions by the light of the lamp that keeps lighting our path.

"Your word is a lamp to my feet and a light to my path."
– Psalm 119:105

This is the path that forever remains on solid, holy ground. Having a relationship with Christ and immersing ourselves in the Bible's words—written as God's love letter to us—give us all we need to live.

Here's my Top 15 reasons to read the Bible daily—chewing on His words, meditating on His promises, and seeking His guidance without ceasing: Gods Word gives us salvation!

1. **God's Word gives us power and faith to apply His Truth to our lives**—keeping us dependent on Christ, not dependent on the circumstances of our disease or disability (2 Timothy 1:7).

2. **God's Word is our line of divine communication**, our unfailing network, to hear the Almighty's voice and respond back to Him through prayer, knowing Christ sits at the right hand of the Father and takes those prayers, spiritual songs, and groans from the Holy Spirit and intercedes (Romans 8:26-27). We can go boldly to the throne of grace (Hebrews 4:16), laying out our requests to the Father

and trusting Him by faith to work in our lives. We know He will always answer our pleas in the way that will bring divine glory to Him, further His kingdom, make His Word known, and grow us and keep transforming us; through the power of His Word, He will keep us cemented in His glory and His will, content even with disease or disability.

3. **God's Word provides the means to throw off sin**, to be like those Christians who came before us (Hebrews 12:1-3).

4. **God's Word propels our on-going transformation, our sanctification**, as we continue to look more like Christ (Ephesians 4:22-24).

5. **God's Word is our guidebook of practical teaching**; through the Psalms, it shows us how to worship, and through Proverbs, it shows us how to live.

6. **God's Word gives us hope and strength** as we endure disease (Romans 5:3-4).

7. **God's Word renews our minds** and as it strengthens us spiritually (Isaiah 26:3-4).

8. **God's Word convicts us when we're in sin and need to repent, and points us back to Christ,** the lit path that will lead to restful elation, life ever after (Colossians 3:2-5).

9. **God's Word gives us examples of how to prevail**, be durable and remain steadfast, under the umbrella of disease and trials (John 14:26-27).

10. **God's Word gives us patience to wait for the return of our King.** (Colossians 1:11-12).

11. **God's Word gives us Scripture to meditate on and speak out loud** when we think our on-going condition or disease is just too much (Romans 5:3-5).

12. **God's Word gives us commands and the supernatural power to not worry**, to not be anxious or fearful (Philippians 4:6-7).

13. **God's Word is our hands-on, always available, timeless prayer manual,** ready to read and pray back to Him (Psalm 23, the Lord's Prayer, Matthew 6:9-23, Psalm 25:1-2, 4-6).

14. **God's Word teaches us how to suit up in Spiritual Armor** to fight against the darkness (Ephesians 6:10-18).

15. **God's Word shows us God's attributes and character** as we love Him more each day and share His message of love and salvation! Knowing His character forever increases our faith, puts our afflictions in right perspective, gives us the hope and peace that surpass understanding, and spurs us on to overflow with faith that draws others to Him as well.

HIS WORD IS . . .

On those days when I'm feeling my most vulnerable, writhing in pain and finding no comfortable position, my body not cooperating and the pain taking over, I can pray to the One who lifts my head.

> *"But You, O Lord, are a shield about me, my glory, and the One who lifts my head."*
>
> – Psalm 3:3

I can rehearse Scripture and pray the attributes of our Mighty God above. I can open my Bible and read the Psalms, and I can worship. I can sing out; I can open my mouth and cry out. I can listen to hymns and worship songs and be lifted by His Truth—the Word that lets me return to Him when He strikes me down in love so that I will know Him in His suffering.

His Word is the rescue mission to the enslaved; His Word is the wind that caresses the plains; His Word is creation's earth-shaking cry: His Word is the brush to the blank canvas; His Word is the cane to the stumbling; and His Word is eyesight to the blind man. I can use the Word to mend my wounds, to bandage my broken spirit, to spiritually give me hope just as I am in that moment. Since the Holy Spirit lives within me, He is giving me the Sword (the Word of God). My mouth can speak words that fight the enemy in combat. The Holy Spirit takes the living Word of God and changes me by giving me spiritual muscles, and I get stronger and stronger. Like a razor-sharp blade, I can wield it; I can use it; I can defend and stab the hater in his black, untrue heart. I like the example of a "spiritual dog" and a "flesh dog"; whoever eats more will be stronger in the fight. We must be stronger spiritually instead of strengthening our fleshly nature. If we are stronger, we are willing to be on the front lines, able to withstand the longest war against this disease.

The Word can also give those around you strength to pray for you when you're too weak or in too much pain to pray yourself. My husband is always praying without ceasing for me. He can pray God's attributes; he can use the verses of the Word of God to give me help, strength, courage, peace, patience, rest, etc. I can always hear my husband's voice as he prays as much as I am feeling the torment in my body during my flare. My husband's voice prompts my heart to calm, and his prayer is my medicine.

We know the Word is inspired, sufficient, and all powerful, so grab hold of those truths, lock them away in the vault of your heart, and guard them. This disease will not steal the Word, and it cannot steal what the Word does for you. Keep your eyes looking out of the high tower, awaiting the light-giving Knight. Disease wants you to walk in darkness, fear, doubt, heartache, torment, and sin, but Christ is the Word, and He will make all new, but until That Day, use His Word to fight—and keep fighting. Our fight is not in vain. His Word will strengthen us and make us stronger. We are not heading into battle unarmed; we are trained by the Word to go into war prepared and armed with the Word of Truth. Be courageous and know His Word holds the power to take no prisoners in combat.

So, let's start the fight. Fight with a satisfied and full heart. Your disease is nothing to the Word of God. Disease will lose every time. In the next chapter, we will focus on the attribute of Sovereignty, so prepare your soul because He is the God of Sovereignty. Praise God! Come quickly, Lord Jesus, come!

Lord,

May Your Word be what we use to combat the wrong thoughts, attitudes, and sin in fighting our disease or disability. May we be strengthened and encouraged by the Truth of Your Word and the way it changes us through Your Holy Spirit. Father, may Your words be the desire of our heart, to grow closer to You by reading them, to find help when we are troubled in our flesh because of disease. Thank You that all we need to fight our sin and temptation is the commands and truths we find in Your Holy Scriptures; may we read them, apply them, and walk away changed. When we face the worst because of what our disease or disability is doing in our lives, give us Your supernatural peace, keep us close, hold us clenched in Your arms, and never let us go. Strengthen our weak prayers and desires and keep us filled with the joyful fight and faith as we live with this disease. When we cry, hear our pleading prayers and wipe our tears away, and may the Holy Spirit use the Word to help us understand and hold fast to You and trust Your will and Your ways each moment of each day we live and breathe.

Amen!

QUESTIONS:

1. What is the Word?
2. Who wrote the Bible?
3. Why is it important to know that God's Word is inspired? Why is it important to know that it cannot change? Can God change?
4. Who is the physical Word?
5. Who is the Holy Spirit?
6. Who makes us grow spiritually from the Word? How?
7. What does John MacArthur say about the Holy Spirit? Why is this crucial and vital to facing disease or disability?
8. What is the armor of God?
9. How does each part of the armor help us fight our disease?
10. What will you take with you on your journey, to remember from this chapter on God's Word?

Chapter Four

CHRONIC CHARACTER AND THE SOVEREIGNTY OF GOD

"When you go through a trial, The Sovereignty of God is the pillow upon which you lay your head."
– Charles Haddon Spurgeon

"Whether, then, you eat or drink or whatever you do, do all to the glory of God."
– 1 Corinthians 10:31

Dear Brave Friend,

Do you wake up to mornings as I sometimes do? On some mornings, I'm the tin man without oil, my knees bowed beneath me like sodden twigs that give way, my swollen joints throbbing, and my bloated body mimicking a blimp in the sky, helplessly adrift. My brain is thick and filled with fog, and I'm walking around on a pier, my eyes fighting through the clammy mist, squinting to see the ship lagging in from a trip at sea. I'm blind to nature's elements, nauseated, dizzy, and can barely hear the foghorn signaling. Does any of this resonate with you? The eyes of my tired heart are shaded, and I'm holding onto my faithful God's promises by a single thread. Sometimes when I'm fatigued beyond comprehension and my exhaustion seems to define me, just the thought of climbing out of bed—my stuffy cocoon for what seems like months—threatens to tax my joints and bones. I watch as my husband pulls out the dreaded walker that I've tried to hide in the back of the hall closet under the coats hanging down from hangers. I've hung them strategically in a precise position, so they casually drape over the unfeeling contraption, hiding it from plain sight, but out it comes no longer incognito.

I try to use it to walk but am still unable to stand and move without laser-beam pain running up and down my legs and gathering around my hips, which indicates my body is just temporal and continues to decay. I find myself having a pity party and pouting, being too proud and foolishly stubborn as I clench my teeth, trying to mask the pain as I attempt to hobble around, barely able to push and feel the movement of the walker's well-worn wheels. I see my husband's face, and he reminds me gently, in a tender, teaching voice that coaxes my tears to stop falling, that the Lord has given me the gift of being "wheelchair mobile."

Say, what? He reminds me that God's love is so sure and so merciful that by being in a wheelchair, I do not have to feel the pain of my throbbing and vexing, broken body. I've never looked at it that way. I understand that God's plan, being only good, offers His best for me spiritually. He keeps me from things that will destroy my spirit, He wants me close, and He keeps me growing. The way He provides in my pain is through offering me the wheelchair.

We reflect on the funny times when I was a backseat wheelchair driver. For instance, in the crowded aisle of Hobby Lobby one day, I tried directing him to grab that one special Christmas decoration, on a too-high shelf he had no idea how to reach, maneuvering through the bustling group of women who seemed to want the exact same glittery angel I'd been eyeing. I come back to reality, awakened from the simple and happy memory.

I return to my doom and gloom doubts and try not to let my imagination take over, but I unhappily succumb to my Eeyore thoughts. I see the future, and I'm not there; I'm gone, my disease raising its arms in victory as the reigning champ. I've let my emotions and anxious thoughts take over. I've forgotten my God's great and pure character.

If you have a disease or disability or take care of someone who does, you probably already know that this chronic health trial is stretching you, and while chiseling away your jagged flesh, it can also reveal a clean, smooth, joy-filled life if you're living by His truths and trust He is your only supply of hope; He is your faithful Ruler. He can take your boulder of trial and shave you down to a nugget of gold contentment if you're walking in obedience as a believer. You need to be reminded that this disease is not only for your spiritual good but that a good God gave it to you, and He will use it to His glory.

The Lord's decisions are always just, right, and true; they're stacked on the building blocks of what His Word says about Him. With disease, you can be assured of His sovereignty and that God can and will use the trial of this disease or disability for your spiritual enablement and growth if you are following and abiding in His Word. The stalks and buds that shoot up from your rooted soul as you settle in the soil of this embedded struggle are not only for you but should be used for the cultivation of your faith and to make an impact on others. What are you saying by your words and actions, and what are you believing and conveying to others in your life if you're walking on air only when life is good and sunny-side up? When life is a sharp thorn that pricks the flesh and goes deep to the plastid bone, and when your sorrows are piling and mounting up like Everest's elevated peaks, God is still good. I want my daughter to see that God is worthy—in the great, in the mundane, and in the unbearable times as well. I want my daughter to see that God is good even with disease. Do you want your relatives, your unbelieving co-worker, your teacher, your physician, your spouse, your children, to see that you love Him and trust Him in every single moment of your given life? His control over your life and circumstances should be the reason you are never anxious, scared, or angry.

We must be filled with His joy and must trust in the living Word by pushing and shoving the Truth back into our hearts when it starts to swell up with earthly doubts that try to seep out through our tired veins and vessels. We must keep following the heart of Christ, not the heartfelt emotions of our flesh. His character does not fluctuate or teeter like a playground seesaw based on diseases, trials, or circumstances. He cares the same and is just as in control, whether you're in ICU for the tenth harrowing day, or in the very throws of battling ISIS in the desert war of Afghanistan, or reeling from the news of a tumor spreading in your husband's body . . . He's in just as much control in heart-sapping, arduous circumstances as He is on the day your first-born daughter walks down the aisle in a cascading wedding gown, or when your son is cured from the very aggressive cancer that has shrunk to nothing overnight. Even though the doctors have taken the credit for and have deemed his cure as a medical advancement and not a healing miracle, you know that God is the One who ordains and directs all. His control does not change, His character does not change, and His sovereignty does not ever change.

> *"God is not a man, that He should lie, nor a son of man, that He should repent; has He said, and will He not do it? Or has He spoken, and will He not make it good?"*
>
> – Numbers 23:19

Your disease or disability is not just a trial for us but for those in our lives as well, and we must know God as good through it. Every morning He is controlling and acting in His perfect character. We must know His merciful love and that His compassions never fail. As each morning the golden sun awakens each creature to see another day, so we are promised one more glimpse of His fathomless, spoken-from-nothing, daylight-and-love gift of life. We are renewed each morning by the promise of His mercies, the mercies that will bring salvation to those who He has declared His treasure, His own in the glory of His will. We must know He is Sovereign.

> *"The LORD's loving kindnesses indeed never cease, for His compassions never fail. They are new every morning; great is Your faithfulness. 'The Lord is my portion,' says my soul, 'Therefore I have hope in Him'."*
>
> – Lamentations 3:22-24

HE IS SOVEREIGN

How can this disease be good? When you understand God's character and view your disease and suffering in the light of His sovereignty, you're reminded that His ways are paramount. If His ways are perfect, then your trial is always good in His purposes as He uses this disease to mature you, grow you, and sanctify you. Knowing His character, trusting Him in it, and following hard to full obedience assures your soul that you will bear spiritual fruit.

"But the fruit of the Spirit is love, joy, peace, patience, kindness, goodness, faithfulness, gentleness, self-control; against such things there is no law."

– Galatians 5:22-23

If you view your disease or disability with contentment, then you will live life in a way that shows you see your entire life, including any and every trial or disease, as part of His plan. Just as you know creation exists because He's designed it . . .

. . . speak to the earth, and let it teach you; and let the fish of the sea declare to you. "Who among all these does not know that the hand of the Lord has done this, in whose hand is the life of every living thing and the breath of all mankind?"

– Job 12:8-10

. . . just as He makes His lightning flash in the sky . . .

"Do you know how God establishes them, and makes the lightning of His cloud to shine?"

– Job 37:15

. . . and just as the skies proclaim the work of His hands . . .

"The heavens are telling of the glory of God; and their expanse is declaring the work of His hands."

– Psalm 19:1

. . . in the same way, you'll see His perfect plan and sovereign hand in the wonders of His creation through the springtime bluebonnets that sprout up in Texas; through the sun's rays that never cease to shoot out like creased, lucent silhouettes across the sky; through the moon perpetually giving off its powdery light; and through the glossy stars you wished upon as a young child that continue to dot the sky like a paint-by-number canvas. You know all these things will happen because He created them.

You know all these things to be true; they are fact, just like His character and autonomy in the Trinity are fact. They are fact because He made them to be, and He controls each of His creations.

"Before the mountains were born or You gave birth to the earth and the world, even from everlasting to everlasting, You are God."
– Psalm 90:2

He is holding your right hand, and He will not let go because He is your Upper-Hand, your Charge, your Ruler and Commander directing you in the troop—a loving General who has no limitation and will never wave a white flag because He dominates and handles the entire world in order and authority.

All authority is His! All the plans for your life, plans that have included disease or disability thus far, all decisions, all choices, all commands are His.

"But who am I and who are my people that we should be able to offer as generously as this? For all things come from You, and from Your hand we have given You."
– 1 Chronicles 29:14

The God who spoke the universe into existence and has given detailed embellishments to the planets, to the universe—to all that He has done—has created all His works with stellar beauty and representation, and He controls all. Let it shelter your heart to know

His design is so much more personal to His adopted heirs, to us, His beloved children.

> *"... also we have obtained an inheritance, having been predestined according to His purpose who works all things after the counsel of His will, to the end that we who were the first to hope in Christ would be to the praise of His glory."*
> – Ephesians 1:11-12

He cares so much greater for His children. He knows every thought before you speak it, and He knows the inner chambers of your heart, your concealed motives you don't want disclosed. He knows the ins and outs of your disease and what is to happen with it. He knows all because He is omnipotent; literally, that means all-knowing. He is in the driver's seat and has plotted the map of His redeemed.

The Bible and our God do not conform to the god of this age. He is not a paper-doll god you can slap a new outfit on based on the season or your personal taste. He is strong and powerful, all knowing:

> *Remember the former things long past,*
> *For I am God, and there is no other;*
> *I am God, and there is no one like Me,*
> *Declaring the end from the beginning,*
> *And from ancient times things which have not been done,*
> *Saying, "My purpose will be established,*
> *And I will accomplish all My good pleasure."*
> – Isaiah 46:9-10

Here, Isaiah the prophet is telling the people to remember all the many feats God has accomplished—from the miracles of the deliverance of His people in Egypt when they were being held as slaves, to their escape at the hands of God through Moses, the stuttering and timid man who became a hero to the people as God worked through him. All the many prophecies fulfilled are recorded so we can remember and give glory to Him; He stands apart and is the only One alone who can fulfill these prophesies.

He alone is God! He alone is God over your disease; He alone is God who can perform miracles; He alone fulfills prophecies. He alone can heal, destroy, build up, tear down, make new, give salvation, protect, strengthen. He alone can enable you spiritually to live as a new creation and throw off the old sin. Remember, like Isaiah wrote to his readers, God is omnipotent, and remember God is omnipotent over your disease.

There are not enough words to encapsulate the adjectives to describe the God of the universe, the Great Shepherd, the Lion of Judah, the Lamb who sits upon the throne, the One who calms the storms, the Horn of my salvation. But there is a key character attribute about our masterful Lord that you can rehearse in your mind to give you strength when you're tempted to sin against Him in your thoughts, words, or deeds, when you are not content with Him allowing you to have your disease or disability. You can choose to be satisfied in trusting His plan and live for Him with this disease or disability because you know He is Sovereign.

RECALL WHO HE IS

Knowing and experiencing God's attributes and character, who He is, shapes how you view your disease. It should stop you in your tracks and make you beat your chest like the publican!

"But the tax collector, standing some distance away, was even unwilling to lift up his eyes to heaven, but was beating his breast, saying, 'God, be merciful to me, the sinner!'"
– Luke 18:13

None of us is worthy, but the One of worth came and made a way, and He gave His Son; He gave you worth. He is your priceless worth, the lover of your soul, the lover of your disease- infested body, and when we think about all He is worth, the eyes of our heart are once again opened. We see the ship coming in, and the fog clears.

Are there days when you feel like your prayers get lost on the way to His throne room, and the fragrant offering rising to the sky that should reach Him turns into a pungent odor that's rejected? Do you ever feel that your words are not heard, that your cries for relief from this disease are dismissed? When these thoughts trouble you, then recall His attributes. Remember that He does not sleep or ever grow tired, that He is always tending His flock like a shepherd.

"Like a shepherd He will tend His flock, in His arm He will gather the lambs and carry them in His bosom; He will gently lead the nursing ewes."
– Isaiah 40:11

Look what else it says in Isaiah 40:28-29: *"Do you not know? Have you not heard? The Everlasting God, the Lord, the Creator of the ends of the earth does not become weary or tired. His understanding is inscrutable. He gives strength to the weary, and to him who* lacks might, *He increases power."*

He does not grow weary, and His understanding is unfathomable. Being a God who maintains these attributes makes him a dependable and faithful God.

We are His bride, and our God is full of truth, justice, honesty, and kindness; He is perfect in His strength, and merciful and full of grace for you in the decisions and the days He has set apart for you. He is not slow in keeping His promise to us about salvation being ours, and He is patient, not wanting any to perish.

> *"But do not let this one fact escape your notice, beloved, that with the Lord one day is like a thousand years, and a thousand years like one day.*
> *The Lord is not slow about His promise, as some count slowness, but is patient toward you, not wishing for any to perish but you the for all to come to repentance."*

> – 2 Peter 3:8-9

He does hear your prayers, and He is walking with you on the bumpy, gravel road of destined trials, forever leading and guiding you to find the quiet stream among the unpaved, dusty path. Those character truths should still your busy and anxious thoughts and soul. You need to know that He holds your prayers cupped in His able hands, and He answers them, sometimes "yes," sometimes "no," and sometimes "wait," because He is doing what is right in His sovereignty.

REHEARSING HIS SOVEREIGNTY

I think back on a vivid memory in my life when someone I knew and loved with all my heart finished her valiant fight with rheumatoid arthritis and its many complications, and she left this earth. She ran this mortal race with firecracker passion for Christ. If you were to look at the bottom of her track cleats, there would be holes burned through the soles of her well-worn shoes. She treated life's competition like a brisk 100-yard dash, sprinting full of love and eagerness to make Christ known in this fleeting, angry world. Each day she stepped up to the starting line in pleasant, antsy anticipation of the official raising of the gun in the air, ready to hear the shot fired.

She used her disease as a gift of Christ to spread His love through her Gospel-centered life. Being in a wheelchair at times only made her that much more eager and readier to see how God could use her. She did not know a stranger, and she could turn any women's frowns upside-down with just one kind smile, word, or Scripture of timely encouragement. As a Christ-like mentor for so many women in our church, she carried the burning torch. I held her close to my heart, and if I could have, I would have given her my heartbeats to keep her here with me. All my prayers, all my desperate, gut-wrenching cries were uplifted to the throne of grace as I pleaded with Christ, my faithful Intercessor, to heal her, even as she was leaving this earth. As I prayed, I was hunched over, grabbing my side, and when I heard the news, my mind spun, my eyes filled with endless pools, and my breath staggered. I was tempted to be angry at Him for numbering her days in a way far too few. "She was gone too soon," I whispered, and was tempted to doubt His plan.

But I knew the character of a God who loves, a God in charge and in full control, who determines our steps.

"The mind of man plans his way, but the Lord directs his steps."
– Proverbs 16:9

I knew that, because of the sacrifice Christ made to give His life for hers over 2,000 years ago on the cross, she was with her nail-scarred Savior when her soul left that hospital bed, and He was the one who had caused her heart to beat and then to cease. No number of beats or thumps I wanted to add would prolong her days; they were numbered, and they were perfect.

"Since his days are determined, the number of his months is with You; and his limits You have set so that he cannot pass."
– Job 14:5

He controlled the beats of her heart, just like He pulsates and energizes ours. He determines in His sovereign, ordained timing when we die and unite with Him if we are His child. I knew because of God's attributes and His teachings in His Word that she was home. She was experiencing a love and holy life that every heartbeat in every chest of every believing soul here on earth longs for. My Christian sister and oh-so-dear-friend left that hospital whole and no longer broken from life's pains. Her body and bones are no longer fragile and cracked like a porcelain doll dropped and shattered. She is whole, not cracked or broken; she is whole!

I can just imagine the scene as she sprinted to the Father's side on her new and glorified legs and as she broke through the positioned tape, lunging forward and crossing the finish line, throwing her arms around Him as He leaned into her and spoke the words we all so desperately long to hear: *"Well done, good and faithful servant"* (Matthew 25:23). Oh, how I miss her!

We can survive those blood-curdling losses and grievous, soul-ripping hurts only by knowing the sovereignty of God. Sisters, this attribute will make our daily labor pangs of life with our disease or disability able to bear. In our heartache, God should be whom we turn to, whom we cry to, whom we worship. Look at the psalmists: they poured out their life to God in song—when peace reigned in the nations, when they were being persecuted and assailed, when they felt lost and lonely, when they sinned and betrayed God, and even during the times when He was silent for 400 years between Malachi and Matthew. The psalmists voice their deep emotions, from psalms of longing and sorrow during the prolonged time God had wiped out entire peoples, to psalms of celebration, praising His creation of the world, to psalms of repentance, worship, forgiveness, and desperation through fear. The Psalms are the psalmists' voices; they are prayers, always pointing back to God. They are never selfish or self-seeking. They understand His tempered control.

We need God when we go through suffering, great loss, the death of loved ones, and diseases; we need Him as a Father. We need Him to put band-aids on our scrapes, we need Him to love us with more than we can humanly understand, and we need Him to do what He knows is best for us. We need to put our life's disease or disability in the care of His character, with the courage and faith to flee the worldly thoughts chasing us; when we find ourselves running toward unprotected realms, we need to turn and run to Him as our Mighty Fortress for safeguard and buttressed refuge, like the hymn "A Mighty Fortress Is Our God" proclaims, a bulwark never failing. When the debris starts flying in our lives, when life's tornadoes bring demolition and loss and sometimes even death to the ones we love, the ones caught in disease's brutal path, He is our safeguard, our strong wall who surrounds us.

Our Fortress is the King of history; He is infinite, in and out of time. His ability to be in control as a Sovereign God is the fact and reality we will talk about, learn about, and meditate on. His sovereignty is unique to Him, not a shared or inherited trait in others; it comes from His spiritual genes and makeup alone, a Father of untouchable character, and it sets Him apart.

Knowing this attribute gives us the mind and comprehension we need to help us understand who He is; it renews and refreshes our minds and thoughts as we know that our disease or disability comes from Him. We should not question why, or how, or when it will be gone. We should not question Him and why He causes us to have suffering, loss, pain, or even death from this condition because, as we will learn, His sovereignty is the glue to repair us when we're the most broken. We are left with cracks, nicks, and gaps, but those are the evidence of how He has grown us, fixed us, and pieced us back together through the many overwhelming and unthinkable woes He has placed in our laps. We are His glued and pieced-together porcelain dolls, carefully fixed with His masterfully utopian hands each time we go through the shame, fear, sorrow, and unkept places of our morose and mournful heart. His able hands and relished devotion for our spiritual advancement fasten us back to Him, and we are even more complete and invaluable, just as irreplaceable and alive as a figurine. His sovereignty keeps us from being that limpid porcelain doll left unaided and companionless, shattered with shards of burnished glass dismantled and scattered, broken on the empty ground. This is not who we are; we are well made, and lovely, as refined china placed in the kiln and emerging even more like Him than before:

> *For You have tried us, O God;*
> *You have refined us as silver is refined.*
> *You brought us into the net;*
> *You laid an oppressive burden upon our loins.*
> *You made men ride over our heads;*
> *We went through fire and through water,*
> *Yet You brought us out into a place of abundance.*
> – Psalm 66:10-12

Here the psalmists are worshiping and celebrating how God came through, even among all the many trials the nation of Israel had endured as God refined them like silver and helped them emerge victorious. This verse teaches hope and shows us His sovereignty over our lives as well.

IN HIS HANDS

It gives us peace to see the world not spinning out of whack like an antiquated spin toy but moving like His masterfully created, seamlessly synchronized yo-yo; when He wants it to spin, it does so in perfect cadence; and one day it will stop with just a quick flick of His wrist. He will pull it up and catch it in His cosmic hand, and it will be no more, but He will create a new Heaven and Earth for those who are His. The Earth will burn, but those of us who are His children will live with Him forever in sanctified, perfect bodies. When someone dies who belongs to Christ, she is home with Him the minute of her final breath, cured, disease free, healed. Amen! Our All-Powerful, All-Knowing is the One—like the elementary Bible song testifies—who has the "whole world in His hands." He is in control of our life. He's got you and me, sister, in His hands. He's got this disease you battle in His hands; He's got the whole world, everything and everyone, in His hands. That song we once sang as children, now that we are older, has profound meaning. Do you believe He has the whole world in His hands? His sovereignty makes Him able to control this yo-yo of a world we live in. So, find your rest and tranquility in His hands.

WHO IS HE?

So, let's find out who He is and what He does, and let's let go of the perceived notions and the faulty view—the ones we hear over and over that have muddled our minds. He is not a Santa Claus God to whom you write a letter, and . . . "Surprise!" . . . Christmas morning, there is the impossible-to-find present you've obsessed over, now wrapped in a shiny, hypnotizing red bow and sitting underneath your piney, ornament-filled tree. He is not like the example that everyone uses of the mythological character Zeus, portrayed in *Fantasia*, who is ready to hurl a lightning bolt down from the heavens if you do something wrong. And He is also not like a fuzzy, velvety rabbit's foot on a rusty, beaded keychain hung from your dashboard mirror, a charm you can rub to give you luck and make your day better. Today's Christianity has turned Him into a roller coaster God, whom you wait for in a long line, jump into in a rush of excitement, and then climb with to the top of the tracks, awaiting the thrill of the loops and skyscraper drops, only to be let down when the car comes to a halt, and finally exiting the ride with a fake Christian buzz.

He is not just one of many ways to Heaven or to eternal life; He is the Way.

> *"And there is salvation in no one else; for there is no other name under heaven that has been given among men by which we must be saved."*
>   – Acts 4:12

He is not weak; or your homeboy; or your only-Sunday God. He's not a popular phrase on a T-shirt. He is the ferocious, stalwart Lion as described in *The Chronicles of Narnia*:

> *"Who said anything about safe? Course he isn't safe. But he's good.*
> *He's the King, I tell you."*
>   – C.S. Lewis, *The Lion, the Witch and the Wardrobe*

He is Holy, reverent and breathtaking. And He controls our lives and plans.

> *"The counsel of the LORD stands forever, the plans of His heart from generation to generation."*
>   – Psalm 33:11

We should treat Him with the honor and reverence He is due:

> *Ascribe to the Lord, O sons of the mighty,*
> *Ascribe to the Lord glory and strength.*
> *Ascribe to the Lord the glory due to His name;*
> *Worship the Lord in holy array.*
>   – Psalm 29:1-2

He is sovereign, and we are not. When you suffer from disease or disability, don't lose your hope. Put your hope in the God who holds your tumultuous health condition in His hands, who holds *you* in His hands, who holds *the whole world* in His hands. Put your confidence in the One who is unparalleled; and let His character enlighten your mind. Give your disease to the One who is over the cattle on a thousand hills, who redeems your life from the pit, whose faultless character will cause us to stand in His presence, holy and blameless, forgiven and free of the diseases that will finally be no more. One of the cures of this disease is found in our God's chronic character of being Chronically Sovereign. So how does that comfort you, my precious sister?

HE IS SOVEREIGN

God retains all rights and exercises supreme and ultimate authority over everyone and everything. In layman's terms, He is over all creation, He rules over all creation, and He controls everything.

It's important to know that, because He is sovereign, He knows and sees all we go through related to our disease or disability. In our human minds, we can think that He is hands-off and not with us, that we are on our own, that everything we do and see happening in our lives because of disease is without understanding on our part, as nothing right is going our way. We can't get a break, we have no respite, everything is backwards, and our hearts can become anxious; our disease or disability is like a broken elevator, moving precariously up and down, never opening its doors, and we keep pushing the buttons over and over with the same effect. It has caused pain both physically and emotionally, not just in our lives but in the lives of those we love and know, like our husband, children, relatives, friends, and coworkers, even with passing strangers, acquaintances, etc. But understanding God's sovereignty should remove your worry, my worry, your stress and mine as well. Nothing is out of His control: you and I can depend on God; He is allowing it. Just look at this verse on how His sovereignty affects you personally:

> *For those whom He foreknew, He also predestined to become con-*
> *formed to the image of His Son, so that He would be the firstborn*
> *among many brethren; and these whom He predestined, He also*
> *called; and these whom He called, He also justified; and these whom*
> *He justified, He also glorified.*
>
> – Romans 8:29-30

I've listed the Scripture references of some key verses below. When you find them in your Bible, you'll discover that each one tells you our God is personal in His care over you, that our personal God has perfect sovereignty over your individual life. Each verse is a relief to our tired soul, when we feel alone and isolated, when we need assurance once more that He stands at the helm, directing and moving in His perfect plan. Each gives you once more the soul-sighing joy that He loves you. My sister, God is in control of you, of your individual life!

- Ephesians 1:11-12
- Job 42:2
- Psalm 135:6
- 1 Chronicles 29:11-12
- Philippians 1:6
- Job 42:2
- Proverbs 16:4

God cares for you. He made all things, and His sovereignty is given to us on a personal level. Having a disease is not a surprise to our all-knowing Creator, and every day that you face disease, He has already planned and carried out that specific day before time. When you close your eyes, the tomorrow that awaits you has already been decided, so rest easy at night and awake joyful in the morning. As believers, we know His sovereignty is His care for us. God's sovereignty is for every person, all to accomplish His purposes in believers' lives. His plans and purposes include not just you, but His past followers as well, as He also cared for them.

The Bible is our heart-resource to let us see the evidence of His faithful control. We can open the scriptures and read about the men and women of biblical times and how He planned their lives. He planned their heartbreaks, their triumphs, their broken dreams, their thrilling escapes, their self-sacrificing deaths, their celebratory births, their lifelong trials, their sufferings, their joyful redemptions, their tearful reconciliations, their narrow defeats. Just as with them, every action and every thought for you has already been checked off your spiritual "to do" list that He created in the life He has for you. It's all to make you grow stronger in faith and keep your character looking progressively more and more like Christ. Here's one of my favorite verses about the grandeur, pith, and power of God working in us, even as we live with disease:

> For in Him all the fullness of Deity dwells in bodily form, and in
> Him you have been made complete, and He is the head over all
> rule and authority; and in Him you were also circumcised with a
> circumcision made without hands, in the removal of the body of the
> flesh by the circumcision of Christ; having been buried with Him in
> baptism, in which you were also raised up with Him through faith in
> the working of God, who raised Him from the dead. When you were
> dead in your transgressions and the uncircumcision of your flesh,
> He made you alive together with Him, having forgiven us all our
> transgressions, having canceled out the certificate of debt consisting
> of decrees against us, which was hostile to us; and He has taken it
> out of the way, having nailed it to the cross. When He had disarmed

the rulers and authorities, He made a public display of them, having
triumphed over them through Him.
– Colossians 2:9-15

Rest easy, my cherished sister!

PROVISION IN THE PIT

There's a person in the Bible very familiar with the control and sovereignty God holds over his life, remaining faithful and trusting in His loving God. As described in Genesis, Joseph is heaved into an abysmal pit, and God knows and allows it; in His provision and protection, He uses Joseph to save thousands of lives, including those of his own family, because Joseph knows God is good.

"As for you, you meant evil against me, but God meant it for good
in order to bring about this present result, to preserve many
people alive."
– Genesis 50:20

He follows when he could have fallen away; he trusts when he could have walked away; he is patient, not in haste; he is loyal in belief to God's promises and in all circumstances, obedient in knowing Yahweh's provision. Joseph is sold into slavery, is accused by Potiphar's wife yet is innocent, and through all his disparaging trials, he knows his Deliverer will abundantly deliver. Just as God rescues Joseph, He will get you through the droughts of pain, the dry and desolate and daily drudge, the impeding blockade or dead-end as your enemy closes in. He is the Ladder to scale that wall. He is your Rescuer, the name that breaks the chains and sets the captives free.

Think of Joseph, who is double crossed by his brothers. Can you truly picture this? As he grew up, the same Joseph who ran and played tag with his brothers and stayed up late with them after bedtime, had a front row seat to the twinkling stars with them as they recited the prayers and scriptures of old, rehearsing the sovereignty of God. These are the brothers he immortalized and longed to be like—the ones he shadowed like an apprentice learning the craft of his mentor; these are the brothers he played jokes on, the ones he would give his life to protect and laughed with after a long day's work; the ones he performed monotonous daily chores alongside and hunted with to provide food for the family. Joseph loved his brothers.

As they grew up out in the wilderness in tents, exposed to any kind of wild animal, they would have trusted each other deeply and loved passionately, but all that changed when Joseph began sharing his dreams. They became green with envy, and their jealously seethed like a locomotive churning on the tracks, never hitting the brakes even as it neared a sleepy town. Can you imagine a sibling hating you and pushing you into a pit, then looking down at you as you huddle in the hole, as you blink your eyes to avoid the fierce sun, putting your hand up to block the crude heat pervading your new confining abyss? Can you imagine throwing your hand up and screaming for release from your new prison, begging for mercy and calling 911 over and over yet getting a busy signal as they laugh, scheme, and then, after walking away, sell you as someone's slave?

What makes this story so interesting is a coat of many colors, a piece of clothing and what it represents: the favoritism shown him through his gift of prophetic dreams, which enrages his brothers yet is given to him by no other than the sovereign God Himself. Because

Jacob, Joseph's father, favors him, they want him gone from their father's loving and cooing protection. They take his tunic back to say he has been eaten by a wild beast, and Joseph hears them planning their acting debut, formulating the rehearsed words they will lie and tell their father. But Joseph does not budge in His trust because He knows that God is the One in control of his life.

When Joseph flees from the wife of his master, Potiphar, and she accuses Joseph of lying with her, Joseph is thrown into prison. The trials that surround him and his pain and suffering look like an endless chasm; but God knows Joseph is imprisoned unfairly. When Potiphar's wife falsely laments, "This is what your slave did to me!" Potiphar's anger burns. So, Joseph is thrown into jail, the same place where the king's prisoners are confined. But the Lord is with Joseph and extends him kindness, giving him favor in the sight of the chief jailer, who puts all the prisoners in Joseph's charge: Joseph now supervises all that happens in the prison. The chief jailer doesn't oversee any of Joseph's decisions because the Lord is with him; whatever he does, the Lord prospers. Joseph believes in the powerful, all-kingdom-owning God, who bulldozes through our human blockades of trials if we obey His Word and put our trust in Him. Even in situations that look fortified like the Great Wall of China, God can penetrate. Whether Joseph's future is filled with more heartbreak, near death experiences, or trials that will bring him death, even if God chooses to give him a disease or disability, he puts his trust in God's mastery and his life in God's sovereign character. God is the One who puts His force of protection around Joseph; and even in prison, God is working His sovereign plan in Joseph's life.

When we feel like we're locked away in a prison of trials, our disease or disability keeping us caged and barred from life without the key to life and freedom, we must remember God's plan never ceases. He is always working. We should and can exude in our trials the same steel, solid trust that Joseph possesses. Joseph knows that if he were to die, or still be under the thumb of worse persecution, abuse, injustice, or torture, he can trust God's tender heart and care over His life. God comes through for Joseph in a way only God can do.

HE WILL NEVER LEAVE NOR FORSAKE US

Just as God never left Joseph, He never leaves you. And he never left Joshua as well, the man who becomes the new leader for his people just before the heroic Moses passes away; when Moses gives charge to Joshua, he lets him know that now, as the people's new leader, he will not only lead them into the Promised Land but will face armies, failure, and ongoing trials; even so, he is to maintain strength in the promise of our warrior Lord's sovereignty.

"The Lord is the one who goes ahead of you; He will be with you. He will not fail you or forsake you. Do not fear or be dismayed."

– Deuteronomy 31:8

In this verse, God says He will go before us, that He will never leave us nor forsake us. Just as God commissioned Joshua and encouraged him, we, too, with disease or disability should withstand and hold the line; we can be heroes in our trials. The courage of Joshua, his belief and stamina to trust God's sovereignty, should give us gallantry to not give up. We can have the heart and faith of Joshua! God was faithful to lead Joshua into the Promised Land.

Picking back up with Joseph's life, we can see God was also sovereign when He restored Joseph to his family, making him Pharaoh's front man in Egypt. Joseph knew God was with him. Joseph the dreamer, who was thrown into a worthless pit like old leftovers tossed in the trash, had become the choice item on the menu. Joseph was never afraid with the Lord as his Protector. We read in Hebrews 13:6, *"The Lord is my helper, I will not be afraid. What will man do to me?"* This verse encapsulates how we should live with disease, knowing He is sovereign, just as Joseph daily looked to His God with trust and was never afraid.

At times, I know you feel like Joseph—like someone pushed you into a boundless hole; deep, dank, bleak, and empty, without comfort; segregated because of your disease or disability; and imprisoned by despair, never to see the soft glow of His refuge like the sun's beams that glisten on the streets after a light rain. But always remember this, my friend . . . you're just like Joseph; everything that happens throughout your life—just as with Joseph—is purposed by God because of His sovereign care and love, and for your good:

> *He sent a man before them,*
> *Joseph, who was sold as a slave.*
> *They afflicted his feet with fetters,*
> *He himself was laid in irons;*
> *Until the time that his word came to pass,*
> *The word of the Lord tested him.*
> *The king sent and released him,*
> *The ruler of peoples, and set him free.*
> *He made him lord of his house*
> *And ruler over all his possessions,*
> *To imprison his princes at will,*

That he might teach his elders wisdom.
– Psalm 105:17-22

God is faithful, and He always keeps His word.
"... which He will bring about at the proper time—He who is the
blessed and only Sovereign, the King of kings and Lord of lords."
– 1 Timothy 6:15

The drought of your disease may or may not ever end, but His enveloped love and having life in Him will constantly replenish your soul . . . it will get you through each moment of your disease or disability; it will be your hope in the downpour of suffering; He will be enough because He is sovereign. He is our soft rain, our patronage after the pressing storm disperses, as the sun bursts through the overcast sky. He is because His promises say He is.

"The Lord is my light and my salvation; Whom shall I fear?
The Lord is the defense of my life; Whom shall I dread?"
– Psalm 27:1

He cannot lie. He cannot go back on His Word. His control is what stays with us. He will bring hope when you are hopeless, faith when you are faithless, a song to your soul when you are spiritually hoarse. He will find you when you're lying in the house of depression, and He is in control when your mind and emotions are whispering haunted doubts that doom the voices of prayer. Let Him have control, my friend, so that these doubts are replaced with worship and spiritual songs pursing our lips, ready to become a melody that keeps us on step. We must be like Joseph and hold our hearts steadfast in love to our Creator, even in the sunless pits, in the heinous times of our disease.

"The Lord also will be a stronghold for the oppressed, a stronghold in times of trouble; and those who know Your name will put their trust in You, for You, O Lord, have not forsaken those who seek You."
— Psalm 9:9-10

EVEN THE WIND AND SEA OBEY HIM

"I have learned to kiss the wave that slams me into the rock of ages."
— Charles Spurgeon

One of the most poignant examples in Scripture of how God controls everything, and everyone, happens when Jesus is with His disciples, resting in a boat at sea. Jesus has decided to retreat to the galley when a fuming storm hits. The disciples are staring death in the daunting face as it approaches on a motioned sea, and they feel prostrate and unprotected. Their minds are swirling with cowardice, the ship rocking. They can't seem to man-handle the boat to steer as they're pitched and flung farther and farther into the open water, into the raven-colored, shadowy tide.

If I can be completely and vulnerably honest, I feel like this sometimes. I want to question Him. I want to mutter words others can't hear, but I still whisper them in my mind, or even say out loud, "Where are you? God, where *are* you?" But I have no right to do so, and the disciples learned this as well. When the disciples make it to the galley of the boat and find Christ sleeping, they hound Him with questions, out of fear, not understanding who He truly is. How can He be sleeping? We know the answer: because He is sovereign. He is the King, the Reigning Messiah, and He is God—even the wind and sea obey Him:

When He got into the boat, His disciples followed Him. And behold, there arose a great storm on the sea, so that the boat was being covered with the waves; but Jesus Himself was asleep. And they came to Him and woke Him, saying, "Save us, Lord; we are perishing!" He said to them, "Why are you afraid, you men of little faith?" Then He got up and rebuked the winds and the sea, and it became perfectly calm. The men were amazed, and said, "What kind of a man is this, that even the winds and the sea obey Him?"

– Matthew 8:23-27

He says one word, and the storm is over. The disciples were feeling as if the storm were the swarthy trial that would bring their end, that they were forever lost in the hostile waves crashing over them, to be drowned, suffocated in the vast body of the high seas. Just like the disciples, we, too, can think things are over. We have one last breath before the water is over our bobbing head; we have lost the life preserver that keeps us afloat out of the storm's vice. If we would stop and praise Him, moved by the power of contentment, and find our joy in the knowledge of who He is—if we would just stop and be still, put on our life jacket, and hang on as we strap in for the choppy sail—we would know that He is always plotting our coarse. He might let us float out into the middle of the ocean, surrounded by only the deep blue, or He could take us into the shark-infested waters, setting our rowboat right in the middle of a Class 5 typhoon—but He is still steering! The hard things show us we were never commanding the boat in the first place. The trials teach us to let Him be the executive Captain, ruling all. The disciples learned about the sovereign Christ, who is over all, as first-hand witnesses. We are taught that the boat is never off balance, unsteady, never out of His reach to put wind in our sails. He is always at the helm, and we are never, ever without our Captain. No storm in the world could ever elude our God's rule.

If God can tame the untamable storm, if He can halt the most dreaded hurricane, the wettest monsoon, the fiercest torch of a forest fire, wild and unappeased, then He can handle my bones and my body. Natural disasters like hurricanes are a gentle breeze; thunderstorms, a sprinkle from the sky; forest fires, a splintered match snuffed out; tornadoes, a spinning fan on low; earthquakes, a shaking maraca. They are nothing and have no control. He controls the things that doctors, scientists, geologists, meteorologists, agnostics, gurus, monks, celebrities, false teachers, and more cannot understand and will never be able to control, fix, solve, reach, answer, or cure.

If we know that He commands the earth and natural disasters, then why don't we believe He has full control over the ones for whom He gave His son? Why don't we believe He controls our disease or disability? With one word, just like in the storm, He can say, "Enough!" and your disease would be gone.

People think that God has no power, that He must not exist if we cannot see His miracles happening and if He is not answering our ever-growing prayer requests and desires. But we know this is not true. We can trust His unchanging ways and His love in designing those plans for us, even a plan that includes disease or disability. We are as beautiful as a well-honed vessel, scratched, discolored, chipped through much use, because the potter sculpted us that way; this is the way His plan is unfolding, and it is real and sure, forged in the light of His marvelous perfection.

AS THE STORMS OF LIFE APPROACH

If we know He is sovereign, then we can trust Him. We accept His sovereignty and His will in our life. Our acceptance affects our actions, our thoughts, our words, our lives; it affects how we respond. If I know God is in control, then I should not sin. I should see sin as an offense, being more mindful of who He is.

He is holy . . . He is the Supreme Portion of my cup that runneth over, His jurisdiction and dominion without beginning or end. When I sin through the way I view my disease or disability, or in thoughts or actions because of my condition, it's an offense to God. He hates sin. He is reverent and preeminent, a truth that should make me more god-fearing and righteous in my behavior, even if I'm sick or have disease or disability. I cannot forget that God has reign over my life. He knows I have a disease; He's not sleeping in the bottom of the boat.

We can see through Scripture that He is imperial; His effectual heartfelt and just authority are not absent in your life at all. God's control is over the most minuscule bug crawling on the sidewalk about to fall into a crack, and in God's desire and control, He directs it to miss the gaping slit in the cement and plod on. His control oversees and guides a baby's first steps. He brought Lazarus' life back from death and swept Elijah up to Heaven in a whirlwind. He let Moses see His glory pass by, and His control with beauty gives patience to a family finally able to adopt the child they've been praying for. It's all in His control. All things are orchestrated by Him. He works out all the details of every being in this world; and in the final, shining kingdom to come, He will be the sovereign, Holy One whom we will worship around the glassy sea.

The times you doubt the most need to be the times you remember His grace—His amazing love and careful safekeeping over your life. When you question if His plan is the best and only plan, you're saying He is not the best, that *you* are. I'm guilty of this, and I know better. A fallen, sinful creature knows better that the universe's Creator? The One who performs miracles, who awoke to tame the sea, steady the boat, and silence His disciples is the One who holds you in His arms and never lets you go.

My friends, even knowing God's loving control, I also know that my disease takes no breaks; it just keeps coming, attacking, proving relentless. This tear-jerking realization, like the sad ending to the movie we know is coming, can make us feel like a boat adrift, our disease never docked. We're constantly at sea, poised and ready to sail out to turbulent waters. The contentment that should fill us lies in understanding the truth—the truth that He forever has rule over the boat and controls our disease. Remember, in one holy word, the storm . . . stopped. I know that when the pain is causing you to cringe, when you feel alone, trapped, pray to Him!

Remember the disciples, and instead of panicking like they did in the boat, ask Him to point you back to the mainland and get you there unharmed. Ask Him to give you His strength; and have faith He will guide you. He will exercise sovereign control over your life. He may eventually return you to port and heal you, or He may not do so on this earth, allowing more pain. Yes, the pain may get worse, the trial may grow more violent, and molasses-thick, dark clouds can form, signaling the doomed storm approaching. But even if so, He is sovereign, always in control. He can never fail us. His plan for your life impacts the world because His will is acting in and out of space in ways that not only affect you but others you know—as well as others you may never see or know. It's like a spiritual spiderweb that includes every human spun into one web. The web affects each insect caught up in it. So it is with God; His ways and will always affect us and always put His glory on display. His sovereignty does not ebb and flow like the noonday tide. His vow does not wash away like a clam stuffed in the coarse sand, only to be whisked back, beckoned by the crashing waves out to the deep. He has exercised all His acts, all His plans before time; they were all sovereignly made.

> *"Thou art the Lord who slept upon the pillow,*
> *Thou art the Lord who soothed the furious sea,*
> *What matters beating wind and tossing billow*
> *If only we are in the boat with Thee?*

> *"Hold us quiet through the age-long minute*
> *While Thou art silent and the wind is shrill:*
> *Can the boat sink while Thou, dear Lord, are in it;*
> *Can the heart faint that waiteth on Thy will?"*
> – Amy Carmichael

THE SOVEREIGN TRINITY

If we know God is sovereign, then we know the Trinity is as well: The Father is sovereign, the Son is sovereign, and the Holy Spirit is sovereign. The God-head, which is three- in-one, are all equal. We have a triune God who is Sovereign. His control over our circumstances gives me great peace. I know His ways and thoughts are higher than mine.

*"For My thoughts are not your thoughts, nor are your ways My ways,'
declares the Lord. 'For as the heavens are higher than the earth, so are
My ways higher than your ways and My thoughts than your thoughts'."*
– Isaiah 55:8-9

He hushes the storm like a kindergarten teacher on the first day of school, quieting anxious children. He has given us His promise that He will never flood the earth again.

*"When the bow is in the cloud, then I will look upon it, to remember
the everlasting covenant between God and every living creature of
all flesh that is on the earth."*
– Genesis 9:16

He has given us His sovereignty, which is His spiritual promise that He is in control. Remember, the stormy trials usher in His spiritual rainbow to our hearts, the promise of His omnipotent character.

THE LORD IS MY SHEPHERD

God has a Love who died for you and came back to keep on loving you chronically; Christ's love will never relent. I can see my disease in the light of His everlasting, forever love, which will endure for eternity. Knowing God's intricate care for each of the billions of people on this planet and even for the children not yet born, knowing He has a sovereign and in-control plan for each one of us, should make us stop and realize that we are not our own, that you and I belong to Him and that He cares. He is your Shepherd, and you are a sheep in His pasture. He provides for all our needs. Just as a shepherd ensures his flock is safeguarded, our eternal Shepherd keeps His staff ready to defend us when the wolf approaches. His arms are ready to carry us out of harm's way, and He does not sleep but is ever watchful and mindful.

"Like a shepherd He will tend His flock, in His arm He will gather the lambs and carry them in His bosom; He will gently lead the nursing ewes."

– Isaiah 40:11

He goes after a lost sheep to bring him into a saving relationship with Him. When a sinner repents, there is rejoicing in heaven:

So He told them this parable, saying, "What man among you, if he has a hundred sheep and has lost one of them, does not leave the ninety-nine in the open pasture and go after the one which is lost until he finds it? When he has found it, he lays it on his shoulders, rejoicing. And when he comes home, he calls together his friends and his neighbors, saying to them, 'Rejoice with me, for I have found my sheep which was lost!' I tell you that in the same way, there will be more joy in heaven over one sinner who repents than over ninety-nine righteous persons who need no repentance . . . "

– Luke 15:3-7

The God who saves is also the God who controls—as well as the God who heals if that is His plan for you. He is a mighty, brave Shepherd who does not sleep, who goes after His lost sheep. At the end of this life on earth, we will be separated from the goats, those who have not repented of their sin and not made Him Lord of their lives. But we who have received His free gift of eternal life and salvation, we with our disease or disability that has made it hard for us on this earth, will be perfected, our bodies redeemed. If God can save the lost, He can walk with you, beside you, protecting you—keeping you as you face your health condition. He will not leave His flock, and you are part of the purposed flock of God's sheep. Rest in the care of a trusting Shepherd!

*So we Your people and the sheep of Your pasture will give thanks to
You forever; to all generations we will tell of Your praise."*
– Psalm 79:13

HIS CHARACTER

Understanding God's character and gaining insight into how you
view your suffering and His orchestration of that suffering will keep
you grounded in Truth, including the Truth of who God is. It will help
you understand how to see your disease as a Christian, to think on His
character, on His sovereignty, when you want to doubt Him, get angry
or anxious, or sin. Remember to see your disease and all you endure
with it in view of God's ratified character, His sovereignty that forever
encompasses who He is. Be reminded of the rainbow and how it graces
the sky, a divine and loving promise, and let it reassure you of His
character. Think on this and pray to the Sovereign One; meditate on
the awesomeness of His character to remind yourself that He loves you,
that because of the Fall, diseases came to be in an impure earth, but
your disease or disability is not a fault or flaw; it's His careful, loving
plan that He is with you and shaping you into the likeness of His first
and only begotten Son. He gave the life of His Son, with a plan that
included torture on a tree, and for you and me it includes disease and
long-suffering, but it will not be like this always. Remember, Christ
is at the Father's side, glorious in His kingdom form, a King with a
scepter who rules in love, justice, and mercy. We, too, will rise and
obtain our glorious bodies when we die.

*"If we find ourselves with a desire that nothing in this world can satisfy,
the most probable explanation is that we were made for another world."*
– C.S. Lewis

WHAT DO WE KNOW?

What can we remember and know because of His sovereignty? His character always gives us hope in suffering because He is in control. I don't have to fear, doubt, or be angry because I don't understand why I'm going through my trials. Remember, we know the sovereign Lord, born in a manger; a sovereign Jesus who lived only 33 years on earth; a sovereign God who was killed on Calvary's hill; a sovereign God who defeated death and surged the earthly mount alive, breaking sin's hold; a sovereign God who ascended; and a sovereign God who now lives in Heaven. God's control was with Him when He was born in a manger as a helpless infant, the same sovereign God whom Isaiah speaks of so powerfully:

> . . . I saw the Lord, high and exalted, seated on a throne; and the train of his robe filled the temple. Attending him were mighty seraphim, each having six wings. With two wings they covered their faces, with two they covered their feet, and with two they flew. They were calling out to each other, "Holy, holy, holy, is the Lord of Heaven's Armies! The whole earth is filled with his glory!
> – Isaiah 6:1-3 (ESV)

He is immutable—unchanging, unassailable, and indisputable—even as a helpless, naked babe out of the womb, and just the same as when Isaiah spoke of His majesty, angels ascribing Him, "Holy, holy, holy . . . !" So, give Him the glory! All sovereignty is His, all control is His! He maintained it in a straw-filled manger, just barely opening His eyes as a helpless newborn, and He retains His control as the Lord God Almighty, as the train of His robe filled the temple with Glory. Grasp that truth that His control is always with Him. Still being God, He could have chosen to drop the cross, to refuse to carry it for us, but He had power over time and knew His mission. He knew His blood must be spilled. If He had control over His life as a baby in the flesh, then know He has control over your life and those you love now. Praise God for His steadfast character. Thank the Lord that you and I don't have to try and control a disease or disability, which we've no idea how to do, that we don't have to control this world and make decisions that affect others around us in ways we'll never see. We cannot, nor could we ever, make the right choices. Because our hearts are wicked, and we are bent on our own ways, it would be chaotic; because we would place ourselves in the center of what we think is right and fair, then our tactics, decisions, and behaviors would mix with selfish desires and dreams, and the world would come crashing down, humanity decimated with sin. We cannot ever know the mystery of His will completely, but we're still called to trust and want to live by His will and not our own. As John Newton said, *"We are sinful creatures who rely on the sinlessness of a Great God to set us free."*

Loving friend, trust in His sovereignty. I have the most godly, wise mentor. She is like my spiritual mom. We have been meeting once a week for over nine years. She has taught me so much as a woman who sacrifices all for the Lord. She faithfully serves the church, runs a Meals on Wheels program, teaches a "Titus 2" Bible study, is always ready to sacrifice for the body of Christ, and meets with me to teach me how to one day become an older woman teaching the younger as she has done for me. She has been there through tears and prayers for my disease, taken me to the hospital and ER several times, stayed with me in the hospital, brought meals to my family, watched my daughter, and been a spiritual leader to me, someone I desperately try to emulate as a woman after God's heart. She always has wise counsel and knows how to keep me going, encouraging me to push open the doors of my trials and walk through with my chest held high, boasting only in Christ. Her counsel is like an antique keepsake necklace that you wear to feel pretty, spiritually pretty. And now I'm giving you, my friend, my most adored necklace for you to wear and enrapture your heart: priceless wisdom, her wisdom. If she were sitting with you right now, she would tell you the exact thing she has buried in my soul, like a time capsule of the most meaningful words you need to hear.

You are like an heirloom vase that God has placed on a shelf, and when He wants you to get it down, He will carefully reach up and grip you in His safe, tight hold and set you down. But right now, in your trial, you're to be content and trust God with the plan He has for you with this disease, to trust in His sovereignty. Like me, God has chosen to place you in a trial where you're constantly waiting on His timing. Like that expensive vase, if you try to get it down yourself, it will break into a million pieces. You must let Him do the work; you must trust Him to take you off the shelf and fill you with the freshest assortment of the floral shop's finest blooms, ones radiating beauty in a June bride's wedding bouquet. And you must trust Him also if He chooses to leave you there collecting chalky dust, used as a spider's sticky trap, ensnaring bugs one by one. Whatever He chooses is His absolute best for you. You must wait and be content to sit on the shelf. You must trust Him and His sovereign plan. Thank you, Penny, for helping me sit and wait on God's shelf.

In all of life, God reigns supreme. In every disease, birth, death, loss, victory, celebration, tear, laugh, word, act, war, political election, surgery, and school classroom and hallway, He is sovereign. On every social media app and website; at every dinner table when people bow their heads to pray, whether that be to the God of the Bible or the god of their own design; at every sporting event, wedding, and funeral; in a storm on a boat; in the darkest of pits; at birthdays and funerals; alone or in a bulging crowd; in America and across the nations; throughout the heights of the heavens to the depths of the bottoms of the unseen saltwater caverns; whether sick or hurt, with disease spreading or cured . . . *He is sovereign.*

He is our Hope, and we can find our peace in His deep-seated Truth, so let your life be lived in His control. Surrender any control you're holding onto by resting in the sovereignty of His character. Your disease or disability is in His control.

> *"For by Him all things were created, both in the heavens and on earth, visible and invisible, whether thrones or dominions or rulers or authorities—all things have been created through Him and for Him. He is before all things, and in Him all things hold together."*
> – Colossians 1:16-17

Praise God! Come quickly, Lord Jesus, come!

THE VALLEY OF VISION

O Lord God, Who Inhabitest Eternity,
The Heavens declare thy glory,
The earth thy riches,
The universe is thy temple;
Thy presence fills immensity,
Yet thou has of they pleasure created life, and communicated happiness;
Thou has made me what I am, and given me what I have;
In thee I live and move and have my being;
Thy providence has set the bounds of my habituation and wisely administers all my affairs.

I thank thee for thy riches to me in Jesus,
For the unclouded revelation of him in thy Word,
Where I behold his Person, character, grace, glory,
Humiliation, sufferings, death, and resurrection;
Give me to feel and need of his continual saviourhood,
And cry with Job, "I am vile"
With Peter, "I perish"
With the publican, "Be merciful to me, a sinner."
Subdue in me the love of sin,
Let me know the need of renovation as well as of forgiveness,
In order to serve and enjoy thee forever.
I come to thee in the all-prevailing name of Jesus,
With nothing of my own to plead,
No works, no worthiness, no promises.
I am often straying,
Often knowingly opposing they authority,
Often abusing thy goodness;
Much of my guilt arises from my religious privileges,
My low estimation of them,
My failure to use them to my advantage,
But I am not careless of thy favor or regardless of thy glory;
Impress me deeply with a sense of thine omnipresence,
That thou art about my path, my ways, my lying down, my end.[6]

Infinite and Omnipotent God,

Our words and actions can never be enough to shout Your loving praises, to recognize the sovereignty that beholds Your beautiful being. Help us to walk in Your sovereignty, to live, breath, and proclaim it, not only to ourselves but to the souls of others. Lord, help us to trust in the utmost care

---

6 "The Valley of Vision." Banner of Truth. https://banneroftruth.org/us/devotional/god-the-source-of-all-good/#.

and affection You have for us and that the disease we have is in Your control. Teach me every day through Your Word about the great magnitude of Your awesome character and Your powerful omnipotence in my life and in everything. You alone are God, You alone are the Owner, Master, and Creator of this world I live in. Let not my heart get anxious or fearful as I know You have me in Your hands. Help me through Your Spirit to find my joy and contentment in You and not the circumstances of this life; and help me to find serene peace in the trust and relinquishment of my disease, knowing You are controlling it when I lie down and when I wake—because of Your Chronic Character and Sovereignty.

Amen!

QUESTIONS:

1. What is the definition of "sovereign"?
2. Is God sovereign all the time?
3. What is important to understanding my disease in the context of God's goodness if I am a believer?
4. Why is that important to understand with disease or disability?
5. How is that comforting to you?
6. What are some faulty views about God?
7. Which one have you been guilty of putting before your eyes as you see God?
8. What are some verses that combat these false views?
9. In what ways was Joseph mistreated? Did he ever stop praising God?
10. How did Jesus calm the storm? What does that tell us about creation?
11. Why is it good that we do not have control over our disease?

12. Why can we trust Him?

13. List verses that give examples of God's sovereignty and the hope each gives us.

Chapter Five
CHRIST OUR CHRONIC WITNESS

"I will keep the ground that God has given me and perhaps in his grace he will ignite me again. But ignite me or not, in his grace, in his power, I will hold the ground."

– John Knox

But I do not consider my life of any account as dear to myself, so that I may finish my course and the ministry which I received from the Lord Jesus, to testify solemnly of the gospel of the grace of God.

– Acts 20:24

Dear Sweet Sisters,

Thank you for reading so faithfully to find yourself here in this book. As you continue reading my open and exposed diary, I hope in the next few pages you can more fully grasp my latest encouragement for you: the disease or disability you're living with gives you the ability to stand out in a crowd, providing a unique way to share with others the comfort from God you yourself have received. Your salvation is your providential bait on your spiritual hook; you can continue to share the Gospel by reeling in unbelievers to tell them of the Gospel's Good News. You can be a shooting star that flashes across the darkness, burning its way into someone's soul. By sharing your story and hope in Christ, and, Lord willing, even helping to lead someone to faith in God's redemptive plan, it won't be someone's wish on a star granted, but instead a "soul-saving wish of life eternal" granted. Use your hope, your story, to be a witness for the soul's saving gift, the salvation for which the disciples literally dropped their fishing nets to run after the Messiah when He called them each by their new names. Use it to call out to people. We are the hands and feet of Christ; we are the voices calling out in the wilderness; and we are the workers for His starving harvest. We hurt with suffering from our diseases or disabilities, and we, like creation, ache and groan at times in expectancy with much anticipation for the shimmering, paved streets, but we are not alone. Christ lived, knowing He would be crucified and sacrificed for believers. We live, knowing our disease can cause us unthinkable hurt, and for some of us, it could take our lives. We have physical and mental limitations, but never spiritual limitations. Living your life with disease is about bringing Glory to His Name. You are loved more than you will ever know, and you can use your disease to sing the song of salvation as you incessantly suffer.

A HEAVENLY HYMN

You are the salvation song if you've been born again by the One the songs in Heaven are sung to without ceasing. You can sing His song here on earth; you are the chosen ballad. Your hymn is made up of yourself and other people, other notes, who will be placed in your living hymnal. Each note, each person you share the Gospel with, makes your song sweeter, richer, capable of encompassing an entire symphony orchestra. These people are the notes we need to bring purpose to our ballad. Listen, and you'll hear the keys that sing, the notes deep and strong, the notes that softly, effortlessly, float as the concert continues—the sounds that move you like the soft creak of a swing in a lonesome backyard; the "swing song" filled with the laughter and giggles of children as the swing rocks back and forth with the hum of the wood as it harmonizes with time. Now the swing sits idle, left alone as time has passed, as each child has now grown and matured, moving beyond the excitement of a simple backyard with a chipped, wood swing that sings its song. That is the rhythm of life: we outgrow the simple tunes, the creaky, white swing. We grow up, but most grow up without the sweet Gospel tune of regeneration. Each note in your hymn is another soul you should bump shoulders and share the Gospel with. Each person in your path, each person within earshot of your joyful notes, can be one you give a smile to as you lend a hand, send a caring card, pay a visit in the hospital, serve soup, and give your time; each person can be one you pray for and share the Gospel with. You should sing your ballad to friends and to family members, as well as to the homeless person you just passed by on the street.

I remember a story of when I first got married; I was in college, and my husband and I were new believers bursting at the seams to be the notes of salvation, to sing our new life hymn, to all within ears' reach. We carried our Bibles on the college campus, and at every break or when waiting to catch the student bus, with our Bible open, we were just begging for someone to take notice, so we could tell them about the One who is "my stay," the One whose voice breaks the cedars of Lebanon.

*"Your lovingkindness, O L*ORD*, extends to the heavens, Your faithful-*
ness reaches to the skies. Your righteousness is like the mountains

of God; Your judgments are like a great deep. O LORD, You preserve man and beast."

– Psalm 36:5-6

We had no money, no fancy home, not many winter clothes; we were "living on love," as Alan Jackson croons in his hit country song. I was sick a lot, but we had each other, and we had Christ. Brad had saved up enough to buy a winter coat as the changing season was fast approaching. I can still remember that coat—a navy-blue wool, button-down pea coat, its shiny buttons etched with an anchor emblem. He looked so handsome in it, not like a twenty-one-year-old kid still figuring out how to live life as a newly married man. I watched from the car as he ran into Subway, the fast-food venue right across the street from our college campus, so we could split a foot-long and, instead of buying a "meal deal," save even more money by eating the left-over chips we had at home and drinking the old lemonade from our beat-up apartment fridge. He took longer than usual, and when he finally appeared, emerging from the doorway to face the winter wind, he was stripped bare of his navy pea coat; it was gone! He opened the car door, teeth chattering, and told me he had given it to a wrinkly, full-bearded man inside who did not have a coat for the winter; he had also bought this man a meal and shared the Gospel with him. My husband was using his voice to be a ballad for Christ. This is who my husband is; this is how he sings his song. This was not a one-time occurrence, either, but how he lives his life and sets the example for our daughter and me.

You, too, can sing. Don't let what you're enduring, your disease or disability, keep you from being someone's tune of salvation. The notes in your ballad should be composed for both male and female, young and old, different races and nationalities. Those in your hometown as well as those in unfamiliar countries need the love and peace of our Awesome Conductor. Your ballad is not your own. If my disease is used by the Lord to save a soul, if I can sing the praises of salvation and be a testimony of the Gospel, if I can share the love of Christ and sing the chorus over and over again, then I will sing that song. If my disease is put on display as the star attraction, and if people stare, ask questions, or need comfort because they are lost, then my song has true purpose. If God has directed my path to cross with those whose song of life is empty and drifting off the pages into an abyss of anguish, like unfinished sheet music that will end in separation from Christ, then I want my song, His song, to reach their ears, to reach every ear of every soul I can touch.

Suffering gives us the ability to use our disease to open the Bible, the heart's Psalms, and pray as God wills it, to let the Spirit come into their soul and awaken their dead heart to a relationship with Christ. The world tells us that we need to be fixed or cured, that our cry of "woe is me!" defines our suffering, but if my daughter is saved because of the example I leave her . . . if I can comfort others through my own hope-filled acceptance of a lifelong disease . . . if my family members see a Truth and determination in me as I hold on to what I believe when everyone else would have deserted the cause, the cause of Christ . . . if my neighbor receives spiritual life through seeds of Truth planted during our "sidewalk conversations" as I hobble outside to get the mail . . . if my disease progresses and my symptoms worsen but, in His sovereign providence, the new doctor trying to find a cure becomes a sister or brother in Christ as I get to share my story while

they're sticking a needle in my vein or going over X-rays . . . then I am
suffering as my Savior said I would:

> *Blessed be the God and Father of our Lord Jesus Christ, the Father of*
> *mercies and God of all comfort, who comforts us in all our affliction*
> *so that we will be able to comfort those who are in any affliction*
> *with the comfort with which we ourselves are comforted by God. For*
> *just as the sufferings of Christ are ours in abundance, so also our*
> *comfort is abundant through Christ.*
>
> – 2 Corinthians 1:3-5

So, sing out loud, sing the song of freedom, sing the melody of
salvation; don't simply whisper or hum your song, but belt it over the
spiritual airwaves as you see it rise and reach the heavens, as you see it
make the deaf to hear and the mourner to dance. Use your suffering to
sing your song. The Conductor is waiting to use your song of suffering
to make you like His Son and to carry the tune of the Gospel, Lord
willing, to all you meet and win their souls for Christ.

PURSUING THE LOST

We all pursue something, and that something is what catches our
eye and our desire; it's what we chase after more than others, hence
the term "pursue." We all know that we get out of something what we
put in. Nike says, "Just do it." Period. That's the slogan—just do it no
matter what. The more we read and study and live like Christ, the more
we're sanctified and the more spiritually mature we become. Just do
it! Look at young David who slew Goliath. Look at young Christ at the
temple studying. Spiritual maturity is not based on age or your earthly
accolades and awards, but on the desire, obedience, and sacrifice of
denying yourself to pick up your cross in pursuit of a loving Jesus. In

our life, we can pursue the pleasures of this earth, the next promotion, the dream of our child getting an athletic scholarship, success, being like the Joneses. We pursue wealth, honor, status. We pursue physical beauty, that outward frame and face that covers the body, which our God intended to age.

Our flesh pursues us. "You need that, you want that," it cries, "Do what you must to pursue and obtain it." Sacrifice your precious, never-enough time with God. Sacrifice your marital duties. Sacrifice your children's spiritual growth. Pursue, pursue, pursue! The pursuit of anything without Christ is vanity, a chasing after the wind:

> *I have seen all the works which have been done under the sun, and behold, all is vanity and striving after wind. What is crooked cannot be straightened and what is lacking cannot be counted. I said to myself, "Behold, I have magnified and increased wisdom more than all who were over Jerusalem before me; and my mind has observed a wealth of wisdom and knowledge." And I set my mind to know wisdom and to know madness and folly; I realized that this also is striving after wind.*
>
> – Ecclesiastes 1:14-17

The more Solomon accumulated, the more he learned that his life amounted to nothing; yet the more he realized he was "striving after the wind," the more stuff he wanted—a vicious cycle that robbed him of a pleasurable life. Yes, he was seeking all the kingdoms of the world except the one that meant all, the kingdom of Christ. No amount of wisdom, knowledge, power, popularity, fame, the charmed life, happiness, answers, world peace, or running after things that take the place of Christ will last. All these flimsy, worthless pursuits and accomplishments will burn. Everything not of Christ that we do for our own self-pleasure and justification, everything we try to pursue that we do and must sin to complete, and everything that is of our fleshly nature will burn when the heavenly alter is lit:

> *For no man can lay a foundation other than the one which is laid,*
> *which is Jesus Christ. Now if any man builds on the foundation*
> *with gold, silver, precious stones, wood, hay, straw, each man's*
> *work will become evident; for the day will show it because it is to*
> *be revealed with fire, and the fire itself will test the quality of each*
> *man's work. If any man's work which he has built on it remains, he*
> *will receive a reward. If any man's work is burned up, he will suffer*
> *loss; but he himself will be saved, yet so as through fire.*
> — 1 Corinthians 3:11-15

Our works will scrunch up and crust over like a marshmallow roasting at a campfire, charred at first, then disintegrating into flakes with nothing but black film left on our fingers. Earthly pursuits are like the sticky white goo from the melted marshmallow, so impossible to get off your fingers, clothes, mouth, and teeth. This is pursuit. These are earthly golden calves. This is pursuit of things that give no eternal security. Boasting in the vanity of self, my strength, my might, my cure for disease, my athletic ability, my knowledge as a CEO, my wit and worth in myself as a godly, has-it-all-together mom—all the things we boast of without our Jehovah Nissi—are just burnt ashes. The Lord God is our Banner, our Victory. Our boasting comes to nothing unless we're boasting in the beat-up Cross and our King who was nailed to it.

We all pursue earthly things at the expense of Christ, and these pursuits are our idols. They are the treasures locked in a chest for which we dive to the bottom of the ocean. The locked chest contains nothing of real worth. As we pry open the rusted box and run our fingers through our pursuits and idols, we realize they're all just fool's gold, hidden there by the "man" who came before. Meaningless to anyone else, they represent a diver's wasted journey. But when we hear about the next booty, circled on a long, lost treasure map drawn up by a greedy pirate with an eye patch and a beard that smells of dead fish, we begin the pursuit again. We want treasure. We dive down for earthly gain when, instead, we could be basking in the sun, relaxing on a beach reading God's Word, and resting in the promised inheritance of our jeweled mansion, plush with the welcome mat from the builder Himself, our Architect who pursued us. The Holy Baby grew up to pursue the teaching of the Gospel to His disciples, and then He pursued death to secure our relationship with Him. Now that's pursuit! I want to pursue the treasures of knowing others can come to Christ, just as He bounded after eternal Life for me with a passionate, boisterous, and Holy pursuit.

NOAH

Noah pursued building the ark and preaching repentance for 100 years before the flood came. Most of us won't live to be that old, whether we're now healthy or sick, and yet Noah preached with vigor and compassion because that's what we're called as Christians to do.

He pursued the calling God placed on his life, continuing to preach and build the Ark, even through mass ridicule, harassment, and daily chiding from his friends and neighbors. But Noah knew an important fact: if those he knew as friends, neighbors, and lost people did not repent, they would be wiped from the earth. And he couldn't bear that knowledge without giving them the Lord's words, warning them to repent and be saved. His love for the Lord kept him pursuing the promise that God revealed to him as the only one on earth deemed righteous. Noah walked with God daily, he obeyed and followed God's laws for his life, and so in obedience, Noah built the ark as God commanded. God took care of Noah by preserving his life and sustaining his family lineage. Noah had to trust God while an entire population was wiped from the face of the earth as the heavens rained down for 40 days and 40 nights, knowing in faith that God would eventually bring back the sun and make a promise of a rainbow in the sky that He would never flood the earth again:

> This is the account of Noah and his family. Noah was a righteous man, blameless among the people of his time, and he walked faithfully with God. Noah had three sons: Shem, Ham and Japheth. Now the earth was corrupt in God's sight and was full of violence. God saw how corrupt the earth had become, for all the people on earth had corrupted their ways. So God said to Noah, "I am going to put an end to all people, for the earth is filled with violence because of them. I am surely going to destroy both them and the earth. So make yourself an ark of cypress wood."
>
> – Genesis 6:9-14

Noah sang the Gospel song every day, over and over. He loved his people and wanted them to fall in love with the supernatural song, God's harmony that sings to your soul for the rest of your days, the song that would save the people from the impending flood that would cover the earth and rid it of wickedness—but no one listened. Noah knew that building a boat would mean that God was going to keep them alive by being shut up in the ark while

CHRIST OUR CHRONIC WITNESS   191

the rain came down; he knew people would drown if they did not confess their wicked deeds. He sang for 100 years, not missing a daily opportunity.

Like Noah, we know the flood is coming—the flood of God's wrath—and we're standing at the entrance of the Ark. It is our calling to keep telling of the Way, the bridge that walks over sin and leads to purity in an old, rugged cross. Sing Salvation's Song to as many as we can, to see them board the boat. Sing! Sing the Heavenly Hymn. Pursue opportunities to sing the way Christ would conduct you to do. Use your life to sing, and don't let your disease or disability hinder you; use it as a tool as you witness and tell people the Good News of salvation in Christ. Disease or disability cannot stop you from singing Salvation's Song and being that winsome witness to others.

FOLLOWING HARD AFTER SHAME

There are men and women throughout the Bible who faced trials, who followed Christ, who received salvation, and who chose the inevitable outcome of death or pain. They chose the shame of the Gospel over the applause of the futile world. They pursued Christ without giving their lives a second thought. Those brothers and sisters who gave their blood, who chose to live so they could die for the sake of the Gospel, who used their own life and their death to reach the nations and proclaim life through repentance, were willing to die for the cause through torturous means. They were willing to face beheadings, crucifixion, stoning, beatings, whippings, starvation, and slaughter because of their love for Christ. This should spur us on to keep fighting!

UNDER NERO'S PERSECUTION

One of the bloodiest of persecutions suffered by Christians was under Nero, the emperor of Rome. During Nero's reign, the saints of God were tortured in the cruelest, most hedonistic and barbaric of ways. Our past brothers and sisters were dressed in animal skins, so they could be ripped apart and torn limb from limb by dogs and other wild beasts. Others were fastened alive on crosses. Some were burned and smoked by the Romans with torches; yes, many faithful Christian martyrs were strapped to poles, doused with oil, and then lit on fire to serve as candles and lanterns to light up the night sky with burning flesh. Nero wanted this torture to be a grand, unforgettable spectacle, so he provided the use of his gardens to display his "Christian lanterns," illuminating his wicked heart and evil hate for Christians and their Messiah.

Others also gave their lives in horrific ways, including Peter the disciple, who was crucified upside down, and John the Baptist, who paved the way for Christ, calling people to repentance, and who baptized the Son, the One on whom the Holy Spirit descended as a dove.

> "... and the Holy Spirit descended upon Him in bodily form like a dove, and a voice came out of heaven, 'You are My beloved Son, in You I am well-pleased'."
>
> – Luke 3:22

John the Baptist moved the people to be baptized as well:
> And you, child, will be called the prophet of the Most High;
> For you will go on before the LORD to prepare His ways;
> To give to His people the knowledge of salvation
> By the forgiveness of their sins,
> Because of the tender mercy of our God,

With which the Sunrise from on high will visit us,
To shine upon those who sit in darkness and the shadow of death,
To guide our feet into the way of peace.

– Luke 1:76-79

And this "prophet of the Most High" served as Christ's devout follower, his friend and brother who also preached, was imprisoned, and then beheaded for the Crucified One. These pilgrims of the faith, our ancient brothers and sisters, were massacred for the Gospel but stood their ground for the God they loved. They let nothing keep them from following Christ. They let nothing hinder their pursuit. Sisters, disease should not keep us from following hard after our Provider, even if we are shamed by the world in our pursuit.

For the woman with a constant, ongoing disease, we have an added struggle; not only are we tempted to pursue those kinds of things that can become earthly idols, but we also pursue a cure, good health, and answers from doctors. We pursue release from and relief of physical pain; it hurts so bad at times that we let that pain affect our life even after it's passed. We understand that the pain will be back because our disease follows us, stalks us, tracks us down. Disease pursues our physical body, our blood, our bones, our muscles, our skin, our immune system, our organs; it pursues us.

So many things we pursue also pursue us. Good pursuits and bad ones . . . such as our sticky-marshmallow, earthly emotions that stay glued to us and become our idol, such as anger, worry, despair, depression, fear, anxiousness, and fretting over those we love; sometimes doubts cling to us, like questioning, "Will I wake up tomorrow?" or "Will I make it through the pain?" or "What if I'm never cured?"

But what we should pursue is help—help from our Creator and His answered prayer that we will wake up from this nightmare, that the clouds will pull back and open, that the God of light will keep us from ever curling up again as the night carries us off to face our disease. We need His help. We need to see that His pursuit is with us in the dead of the night, that His pursuit turns the dark into light. He is the Hope of the morning sun that will awake us. We can see the sunrise if we will pursue Christ. God does not want us to be sad, fearful, or anxious, but to trust Him, choosing to live this life in complete trust of Him with our disease or disability. God has given us joy amidst the affliction. Be that kind of bright light for others! May we pursue Christ like He pursued us. May that be our holy pursuit; may that be our mission.

SANCTIFICATION

We also need to pursue sanctification, thankful for the sacrifice God gave us in redeeming us. When we are saved, we are sanctified—set apart from the world and unto the Lord. At the exact moment when you are saved by grace, your conversion takes place, and you are positionally sanctified.

> *"Or do you not know that the unrighteous will not inherit the king-dom of God? Do not be deceived; neither fornicators, nor idolaters, nor adulterers, nor effeminate, nor homosexuals, nor thieves, nor the covetous, nor drunkards, nor revivers, nor swindlers, will inherit the kingdom of God. Such were some of you; but you were washed, but you were sanctified, but you were justified in the name of the Lord Jesus Christ and in the Spirit of our God."*
> – 1 Corinthians 6:9-11

You have a Holy standing in Christ through faith. It's Christ who has done the work in us. This work is past tense because the moment of our spiritual birth, we are holy. In God's eyes, He sees us just as Holy as Christ. Our position in being like Christ is nothing we have done. In short, positional sanctification is our right standing before Christ the moment we are converted, the minute God gives us salvation. But our sanctification continues while we're here on earth and ultimately will consummate when we reach Heaven. May our mission be to become more and more sanctified in the Truth!

Progressive sanctification is the process of becoming more like Christ. It's how we should pursue Christ; it's our obedience. In positional sanctification, Christ does the work, but in progressive sanctification, we put forth the obedience and effort to grow in looking and becoming more like Christ.

"For those whom He foreknew, He also predestined to become conformed to the image of His Son, so that He would be the firstborn among many brethren."

– Romans 8:29

We are called to kill our sin daily. We must every day mature in Christ by dying to our sin. How? By becoming like our Master, our Sin Slayer, the One who bruised the serpent's heel. It's imperative that you grow in your progressive sanctification as you face your disease head on. So, look at this list and begin designing your life around the Truth and logistics of these means. We pursue being conformed to Christ's image as conveyed in Romans 8:13: *"... for if you are living according to the flesh, you must die; but if by the Spirit you are putting to death the deeds of the body, you will live."*

Reading and memorizing God's Word. 2 Timothy 3:16-17, Psalm 119:15, Deuteronomy 11:18, Psalm 37:31, Proverbs 6:2, John 17:17, Proverbs 3:3-4, Psalm 1:2.

Praying. 1 John 5:14, Psalm 17:6, Romans 12:12, Matthew 6:9-13, Philippians 4:6.

Obeying God's commandments. Deuteronomy 11:1, John 14:15, 2 John 1:6, Luke 11:28, James 1:25.

Growing through trials as we trust Him. Proverbs 3:4-6, James 1:2-4, John 14:27-28, James 1:12, Romans 12:12 Romans 5:3, Romans 8:18, 1 Peter 4:12.

Giving glory to God in all we do. Psalm 9:1, Colossians 3:17, Psalm 28:7, 1 Thessalonians 5:18.

Living out His truths and promises. Philippians 4:9, Ephesians 5:8.

Being a witness for Christ and sharing the Gospel. Matthew 5:16, Philippians 2:14-16.

Being a living example of a follower of Christ—even if we are sick and have a disease. 1 Timothy 4:12, 1 Peter 2:21, Ephesians 5:1-2, Philippians 2:1-8, James 2:14-17.

We need to continue our pursuit of looking like Christ. We need to continue through our progressive sanctification. We will always have sin because we are fallen, but as my pastor says:

"We should have a decreasing pattern in our sin and increased pattern in holiness."

– Tom Pennington

People who are preparing and blazing the trail for their urgent, heartfelt pursuits have put the time, energy, resources, and heart into what they believe and follow. When we get married or have a relationship based on Christ, it takes careful preparation to be ready to go "all in." Just as man is a vapor, a flower that will blow away, we must use all are days to His glory:

> *As for man, his days are like grass;*
> *As a flower of the field, so he flourishes.*
> *When the wind has passed over it, it is no more,*
> *And its place acknowledges it no longer.*
> *But the lovingkindness of the LORD is from everlasting*
> *to everlasting on those who fear Him,*
> *And His righteousness to children's children,*
> *To those who keep His covenant*
> *And remember His precepts to do them.*
> – Psalm 103:15-18

Like dandelion dust blowing in the wind, our time on earth is short, making it so exceptionally vital to pursue Christ in all we do in this mortal life. God never hesitated to pursue us and give us salvation and then use the Holy Spirit within us to help us pursue godliness. God went "all in," and we're called to do the same. Yet, we're called to do so differently than other people surrounding our inner circle; we're called to pursue Him even with having disease or disability.

ACTIONS FOR CHRIST

Some people with disease or disability are unable to attempt what others would consider major witnessing feats, but every time you share the Gospel with the right heart and attitude in Christ, it's a sacrificial accomplishment; we're not doing it in our own strength but to let the Holy Spirit work through our weakness. When we share the Gospel, we're being obedient and compassionate, merciful and sacrificial, to want to see God's Spirit open their hearts to regeneration, save their souls, and escape Satan's forever torment. We can always stand for Christ by the choices we make to honor and praise His name. If we are physically unable to do so at times, then we can trust that the Lord always accomplishes His will. God doesn't need us, but He can use us when we bow the knee, when we desire to see His kingdom go forth and others to come into a saving relationship with Him.

> *"We must make the invisible kingdom visible in our midst."*
> – John Calvin

In any trial, we can do the most important thing: we can be obedient to what the Bible teaches, and we can pray. We should pray for God's will, for strength, and for others who are sick or persecuted, who are lost and haven't received baptism into New Life. We should pray for their salvation. We should pray for a sound mind and a bold voice to share the Gospel; for wisdom in a world where the masses are willing to sell their soul for applause from mere mortals, for trinkets and treasures that moths and rust destroy.

> *"Do not store up for yourselves treasures on earth, where moth and rust destroy, and where thieves break in and steal. But store up for yourselves treasures in heaven, where neither moth nor rust destroys, and where thieves do not break in or steal."*
> – Matthew 6:19-20

Pray that the Lord can use you with your disease. We can be just like these Christians who lived before us; we, too, can choose to honor Christ no matter what our diseases bring us—no matter the circumstances, trials, and setbacks that besiege us. We know God can use our life and disease to promote and further the Gospel. The urgency to further the Gospel is great, especially in a generation that has washed their hands as Pilate did and will continue to hand Christ over and over again to be crucified. We have the Scripture to place our faith in and teach us to live with an abundance of deep peace and joy, even in this "carnival world" that will sell you a soul-priced ticket for a ride that leads straight to Hell. But as Christians, our ticket is an eternal pass to the life of the supernatural realm of Heaven, the ticket that secures our stay, because we followed hard after His name and the shame of the Gospel.

JESUS, OUR SUFFERING SAVIOR

In the Bible, the One who suffered the ultimate punishment for us never needed any rescuing. In fact, the One who suffered did the rescuing. See Galatians 1:3-4 and 1 John 4:10, as well as this Truth: *"For even the Son of Man did not come to be served, but to serve, and to give His life a ransom for many"* (Mark 10:45).

May you know God's peace. As you suffer, use *your* suffering to rescue, use your pain to win hearts, use your disability to show the perfectness of a Father who has made you. Suffering can be a tool for you to tell other souls about Christ. In all of Scripture, we're never taught that we will live our best life now; we are never taught to be purpose-driven about ourselves; we are never taught to make ourselves comfortable but to be uncomfortable. We are never taught to be *of* the world but simply *in* the world. We are taught by our Christ that because the world hates Him, it will hate us as well, and that if He was persecuted in this world, then we also should expect persecution.

*"If the world hates you, you know that it has hated Me before it
hated you. If you were of the world, the world would love its own;
but because you are not of the world, but I chose you out of the
world, because of this the world hates you."*
— John 15:18-19

Today and every day as a follower of Christ, we must be willing
to be flogged, whipped, and spat upon as we brave Calvary's hill
and feel our own flesh nailed to the wood. As we cry out, we will
not be silent about the Truth of God's Word but be willing to suffer for sharing it. We must be willing to suffer because the world
brings suffering, but Christ will always bring satisfaction in the
life to come.

A MARTYR

In Scripture, we learn about a man named Stephen, the first
martyr. Stephen witnessed the heavens open, and he was stoned
for speaking the Gospel. I cannot imagine the terror of standing
before an angry mob hurling rocks at me, to have to take those
excruciating blows of flint puncturing my flesh and pounding
my bones, and yet Scripture records that, as he was being stoned,
Stephen looked up. He looked up because his Father opened the
Heavenlies to embrace his bloody body and welcome his now pure
white soul. Stephen suffered. Prior to his stoning, Stephen shouted
out to the people in court, standing trial for justice for the creed
of Scripture:

*Now when they heard this, they were cut to the quick, and
they began gnashing their teeth at him. But being full of the Holy
Spirit, he gazed intently into heaven and saw the glory of God, and*

Jesus standing at the right hand of God; and he said, "Behold, I see the heavens opened up and the Son of Man standing at the right hand of God." But they cried out with a loud voice and covered their ears and rushed at him with one impulse. When they had driven him out of the city, they began stoning him; and the witnesses laid aside their robes at the feet of a young man named Saul. They went on stoning Stephen as he called on the Lord and said, "Lord Jesus, receive my spirit!" Then falling on his knees, he cried out with a loud voice, "Lord, do not hold this sin against them!" Having said this, he fell asleep.

– Acts 7:54-60

Will we speak the Truth even with the degree of agony we're in? Will we be faithful to trust as Stephen did, even if men pick up stones to bludgeon us as they did him? Are we willing to keep undergoing the fatigue that disease causes our heart? Are we willing to further the Gospel with our disease just as Stephen furthered the Gospel with his innocent plea and objection to the lies, with his willingness to tell the Truth of the God-man who loved him, to sing out the Truth, knowing it would cost him his life? Beloved sister, will you be the Truth? Can you suffer for Christ, knowing it's His plan? Can you take the torture of disease and still love the Great Physician? In Christ we can, in all circumstances. Can you be content in life with the thorn that plagues you? So, remember, my bold friend, be a rescuer in your suffering. Belt out the tune of salvation.

LOVER OF MY SOUL

For some of you, your disease has reached a place where you are bedridden, or in the hospital receiving another infusion, or in the hospital right now indefinitely. Perhaps you've been moved to assisted living. Or it's time to begin your last vestige on this earth, your last remaining days in hospice. Maybe, today your sweet quadriplegic child is having complications. With anxious anticipation, perhaps your loved one is in so much anguish that this could be the time the Lord calls him home to see the Savior, the Suffering Servant face-to-face. God did not give us a permanent longing to want to live here forever in a tarnished world, one that chips like an old trophy, with the gilded plastic and painted gold flaking away, revealing only a fake existence. God did not give us the desire to want to remain here in a broken-mirror world that has progressed from a hairline crack into sharp fragments that break and pierce our hearts. He gave us that longing, that overwhelming desire and ache, for our hearts to be with His in Heaven—welcoming us, opening the front door, and having us sit down at the banquet, the party He is throwing in our honor, where He will serve us and there will be no more suffering.

So, hang on and keep singing the Gospel ballad! Ponder on your suffering, reflect, meditate on it, and then look up Scripture to comfort you. I pray you understand that enduring the suffering of disease is part of the trial in your life that God has used to make you more like Him and to bring you into a closer relationship with Jesus. I hope you will seek the counsel of the Lord's Word, and I pray you have silenced the out-of-tune song within your heart to, instead, sing the hymns of praise He is due. In this life, I've found that the more I suffer, I can do one of two things: First, I can praise Him for this trial and let the Spirit teach and mold me to have a joyful and willing heart; I can love the Lord with all my heart, soul, mind and strength; I can find my contentment in my disease; I can be silent and know that he is God.

Or, second, I can push away from Him in anger and bitterness and let my sphere of life become filled with idols as I start to rot away like a dead, half-eaten animal. We do not have to let our sin cause us to rot; we can be content. He is our contentment!

Suffering binds our hearts and entwines our souls. We must realize that our beating hearts are not given to us to serve our selfish agenda, but to fulfill His Sacrificial Purpose. Our song is not ours, but the Lord's. I want to thrive in God's love and mercy; I don't want to rot away to be picked up by buzzards, but that's what it feels like when I'm in sin. Until you repent, your soul and heart can start to rot—I know this feeling. We can realize that we have this disease with Him as our Master and the Lover of Our Soul, or if we don't know Him, we can live this life with disease or disability without His guidance, comfort, and hope, completely on our own and doing things our way until our last day on this earth when we meet him, not as our Savior but as our Punisher. Yet, for those who know Him and trust Him, we know that as we suffer, He is our song; as we suffer, He is with us.

I know we don't know each other personally but know that I'm still your friend, your sister who can—either in some small or ginormous way—sympathize with you. May God use your heart hymn and keep conducting you with all mercy and all grace. He can do no less; He can only do perfection, and those aches and pains are not in vain. They are just one of the verses that makes up your redemption ballad—the song you are ready to sing! Praise the Lord, come quickly, Lord Jesus, come!

"When God calls a man, He does not repent of it. God does not, as many friends do, love one day and hate another; or as princes, who make their subjects favorites, and then afterwards throw them into prison. This is the blessedness of a saint; his condition admits of no alteration. God's call is founded upon His decree, and His decree is immutable. Acts of grace cannot be reversed. God blots out His people's sins but not their names."

– Thomas Watson

Father in Heaven,

We are weak without You; we need You working in us through the Spirit, the One You left with us as our Counselor, who lives within us. Disease and disability should not hold us back from witnessing and sharing the Gospel with others. Help us to be brave to sing the Gospel tune. Help us to not fear the world's persecution and help us to want to put others before ourselves. Lord, we want to do so much for Your kingdom, but what You require is that we love You, serve You, and be obedient to Your Word. Help us to know that nothing we do can bring salvation into the hearts of men; we are just called to be Your tool and ambassador. You're the One who opens the heart and help us in our weakness to have a desire to see hearts opened as we share the love of Your Son, as we share the Truth of His sacrificial death on the cross, for all those who would repent and make You Lord of their lives. Make us bold like John the Baptist to preach repentance and the Good News to all You bring into our lives. In Christ's name, amen!

QUESTIONS:

1. What is the Gospel? Write it out using Scripture so that you will be ready to share with others.
2. What is sanctification?
3. What is positional sanctification?
4. What is progressive sanctification?
5. When will we truly be sanctified?
6. What are some idols you pursue?
7. What can you do to eliminate those idols in your life?
8. Who comes to your mind who needs salvation? Think of someone you can begin praying for. Pray for opportunities to share the Gospel and be a witness for him or her.
9. Who preached for 100 years? Why? Do you have that kind of desire to see others know Christ?
10. Write out some ways you can be bold for Christ.

Chapter Six

CHRONIC SUFFERING WITH ENDURANCE AND CONTENTMENT

"God has chosen not to heal me, but to hold me.
The more intense the pain, the closer His embrace."
– Joni Eareckson Tada

He was despised and forsaken of men,
A man of sorrows and acquainted with grief;
And like one from whom men hide their face
He was despised, and we did not esteem Him.
– Isaiah 53:3

Dear Suffering Friends,

As coheirs with Christ, we're often presented with some common questions from non-believers, those without faith in Him; they sometimes present arguments that ask why a "loving" God would, in their words, "make" suffering. God did not make suffering; suffering was a consequence of the sinful acts man committed by choosing his own will, his own selfish desires, acting on the pride of his heart. For instance, when Adam and Eve ate of the fruit in the garden, their eyes were opened, not as God's eyes see and know all, as the serpent promised, but as exposed children who were afraid and hid. They both realized they were naked. They sinned, and the consequence of their sin would produce suffering in their lives as they were banished from the perfect garden and forced to live apart from God.

As a Christian with disease, I have read about suffering all through the Bible. I have seen disease and sickness like a painful hangnail; it's everywhere and never at a place where it can cease throbbing, even after you try to file it down. I have seen it in my life, in my friends' lives, and in the unnamed faces I sometimes see but will never know. I see starving, bony, saggy-eyed children with dirty, dusty, infected feet, carrying malaria, with ribs sticking out of their tiny frames, who were born in remote countries. I see children who make their way into the cancer treatment centers, their parents carrying suitcases while the child clutches his blanket and favorite worn-out stuffed bear, about to begin the fight for his young life. Like a rusty nail that punctures soft skin and leads to deadly infection, disease and suffering cover this world like moss on a roving river rock. Disease and disability are universal, and because Adam and Eve took a bite of the forbidden death fruit that forced disease, suffering, sin . . . and it all entered the world:

> When the woman saw that the fruit of the tree was good for food and pleasing to the eye, and also desirable for gaining wisdom, she took some and ate it. She also gave some to her husband, who was with her, and he ate it. Then the eyes of both of them were opened, and they realized they were naked; so they sewed fig leaves together and made coverings for themselves.
> – Genesis 3:6-7

As humans, we will never fully grasp and understand why people must suffer, because suffering can entail horrific, graphic details. We are sometimes witnesses to the ones we love experiencing the brunt of suffering's taunt. It's far beyond our comprehension and tiny brain to fathom the God of the universe and the plans He has designed for us when they include persecution, pain, suffering, and death too soon. But those aches and pains are not in vain. We can depend on our Savior by enduring as He did.

So how do we endure our suffering? Our dependence is not a wait-and-see attitude; it's a mobile force. We're not called to a slack faith. Look at this verse in James, describing how we should face trials:

> *Consider it all joy, my brethren, when you encounter various trials, knowing that the testing of your faith produces endurance. And let endurance have its perfect result, so that you may be perfect and complete, lacking in nothing.*
>
> – James 1:2-4

Faith produces endurance. So, what is endurance?

WE CAN ENDURE

Endurance is an interesting word. The dictionary defines endurance as "the fact or power of enduring an unpleasant or difficult process or situation without giving way," as in, "She was close to the limit of her endurance." Yet, when I hear this definition, I'm disgusted. "Unpleasant or difficult"? Our circumstances are so much, much more than unpleasant and difficult, and endurance is not a "process" to someone who has a disease; it's our daily reality. It's a huge and defining part of our life, but our endurance in the trust of Christ is greater! Our world tosses the term around so loosely, like a backyard pickup game of football between a couple of dads getting together to relive their glory days. "Endurance" is nothing that should be tossed around. We hear examples of a football team showing stamina and endurance to make it through the game's four quarters. Others remark how they show endurance by exercising: walking, biking, running, swimming, hiking, and even dancing are considered endurance exercises. Endurance is getting your heart rate up while you work out. Endurance is given a superhero name if you're a good athlete. It's like being an Olympian or running a marathon—all those people show noble endurance. We look up to people in this world who show grit and tenacity. Endurance is synonymous with athletes, and athletes today make millions of dollars for being able to show off their gutsy ability to spiral a football down the field, pitch a no hitter in the majors, win a gold medal in the Olympics for jumping the final hurdle in the steeple chase, or shooting a game-winning buzzer beater in Madison Square Garden to a sell-out crowd. Our world can place too much emphasis on that kind of endurance.

Biblical endurance is different. The determination and stamina we possess do not come from trying to muster up our own strength. If you are in Christ, they come from the Lord and His strength. We depend on Him to give us our fortitude:

> *The Lord is my strength and my shield;*
> *my heart trusts in him, and he helps me.*
> *My heart leaps for joy,*
> *and with my song I praise him.*
> *The Lord is the strength of his people,*
> *a fortress of salvation for his anointed one.*
> – Psalm 28:7-8

Having a continually active disease is having endurance. My former Titus 2 Bible study leader battled an aggressive cancer, and she reflected the resilience of Christ until her body gave in and her soul left to be at His side. She taught many of my good friends and I how to be hospitable, loving, and serving wives; she reminded me so much of Tabitha in the Bible. She endured with grace, trust, and dignity for Christ and the plans He chose for her.

> *"In Joppa there was a disciple named Tabitha (in Greek her name is Dorcas); she was always doing good and helping the poor."*
>
> – Acts 9:36

I had a dear sister in Christ who showed endurance. She's the one I've mentioned before, and she encountered many surgeries to put steel pins in her hands and feet because of what the rheumatoid arthritis was doing to her body, yet she never hesitated through all the pain to bend down and pick up one of her grandkids when she would see them running down the hall in the church foyer. Her tenacious belief and fortitude in her trial never wavered; her gallantry with joy fizzed like a shaken soda can. She taught me so much. She helped me endure for Christ. She was a teacher, and I was a student in the class she taught: "How to Endure Disease with Christ."

In "Chronic Endurance 101," I sat at the front and listened eagerly, taking in the knowledge and wisdom as she wrote on the chalkboard of life, 'til God called her home. I cannot wait to see my dear sister on the streets of gold as she walks with grace and beauty, strolling and skipping, her steps no longer wobbly, her body no longer confined to the smooth, steel of a wheelchair as she was at times, but instead enjoying a complete and healed body, unequaled and marvelous, smiling and worshiping. We will be there one day, my friend, if we keep enduring, so get to class early and let the Teacher of the Heavens instruct you. Bring your sharpened pencils, take endless notes, and stay after for tutoring. He will teach you and me how to endure because the answers are at our fingertips: our answer is His Word.

"My soul is weary with sorrow; strengthen me according to your word."
– Psalm 119:28

I know a man diagnosed with terminal cancer, not once in his life but twice, and he endures radiation and the horrific side effects every day. Still, I see his kind and gentle face singing praises in the choir every Sunday to the God who has stricken him with a terminal brain tumor; that is godly forbearance.

I know a college girl who was on the diving team, and now, instead of her jumping off a diving board, twisting her body into a graceful flip, and waiting for the judges' score, God has given her a PICC line, as well as shocking pain from multiple diseases. She shows jubilance and a resolute backbone, and she loves Christ so much that her life is the Gospel lived out in word and deed; that is steadfast faith in Christ.

Perseverance is the middle-aged wife who now lives with her spouse undergoing in-home healthcare, helping him with his self-care needs like brushing his teeth, combing his thinning hair, and tending to all his hygienic needs, as well as directing him in everyday tasks. She is exhausted by the end of the day but still rises early each morning to open her Bible and start the day with time before the Lord. She loves her husband just as much today as when they walked down the aisle, now honoring her vow before the Lord to love each other in sickness and in health.

My pastor's wife is a woman of gracefulness and esteemed character. While she is tall and stunning in looks, her presence is felt when she walks in the room, not because of her appearance but because of how her character speaks to others. She has an autoimmune disease and has battled cancer as well, but she is still the epitome, the gold standard, of what a Proverbs 31 and Titus 2 woman looks like.

Each one of these examples are people I know and love. These heroes of mine are who give me hope to endure through their biblical love of Christ and commitment to persevere; they trust God, and they show every day that their life does not belong to them but to Him. These beautiful children of God are the strong pillars of endurance and faith who support and keep the example of godliness in the middle of tender and heart-tugging trials.

In my own personal journey, when the pain is at its worst, I still have a hope, a peace that He gives me. I know His Word is true. I know His love and His promises will sustain me. I know I can live moment by moment, day by day—just as He will help you when you are weak as well. As you go through your days filled with pain, do not grow weary.

"Consider him who endured such opposition from sinners, so that you will not grow weary and lose heart."

– Hebrews 12:3

Instead, know that He promises to sustain you spiritually if you're walking and living His Truth.

Just look at these examples in the Bible: God sustains Elijah by sending an angel to give him food, and Elijah endures while he waits (1 Kings 19:7-8). God sustains Daniel, who was left to be mauled in a den of lions, left for dead with no way to defend himself (Daniel 6:19-21). He sustains Christ in the wilderness as Satan tempts Him, and He endures the temptation (Matthew 4:8-11). He sustains the young, pregnant Mary as inside her womb she carries the Creator, Christ our Messiah; and He sustains Joseph, her loyal and determined husband as they endure their long peregrination, their arduous journey to Bethlehem (Luke 2:3-5). He also protects them from Herod, the king who planned mass genocide of all babies under two years old (Matthew 2:13-15). By doing this, He kept Jesus, His Son, alive and sustained; by doing this, He fulfilled the ultimate plan, the Gospel, so that we today as followers can "go and make disciples" as we share the Good News.

He sustained each of these forerunners to our lives of faith, through the most dangerous and perilous of times, and He will sustain you if you trust in Him through the pain of your disease or disability. Reread these examples along with the Scripture verses, and remember once more how God rescues, shelters, sustains, provides. Let the Word of God soothe your soul and strengthen you in these times when your heart is vulnerable and shaky.

SAUL TO PAUL

Paul suffered and recounts his sufferings in Scripture, but he also acknowledges that he doesn't fully comprehend, does not get 100 percent, all the reasons for his pain-filled trials, but still, he accepts them. Even with all his godly wisdom, he admits he could never know God's ways. And this is the answer; this is the key to understanding! We don't know God's ways . . . but we don't have to anyway. We can trust Him regardless! In Romans 11:33, Paul says, *"Oh, the depth of the riches of the wisdom and knowledge of God! How unsearchable his judgements and his paths beyond tracing out."*

This is a man who knows suffering. If anyone has reason to want to walk away from God and turn his back on the Christian faith, it's

Paul. And Paul isn't one-and-done with suffering; it follows him like a lost puppy, nipping constantly at him through the thorn in his flesh. After Paul asks God three times to remove the thorn, and God chooses not to do so, Paul still can say that God's grace is sufficient.

> *Concerning this I implored the Lord three times that it might leave me. And He said to me "My grace is sufficient for you, for power is perfected in weakness." Most gladly, therefore, I will rather boast about my weaknesses, so that the power of Christ may dwell in me."*
> – 2 Corinthians 12:8-9

We don't really know what the thorn is. Commentators think it could be his eyesight, a physical ailment, or even persecutors of the church who would just not leave him alone. Whatever its source, it's heavy enough and all-consuming enough to bring Paul so much grief that he cries out to the Lord and implores him three times. The definition of "implore" is to beg or beseech. Paul begs the Lord; he literally pleads and sets himself up in a vulnerable state to humble himself to beseech God.

Consider a homeless person on the street with no daily morsels, someone desperate enough to emblazon a piece of cardboard with "Will work for food." Indeed, that person is begging, not caring what anyone thinks and willing to do anything to have just one scrap, one meal. Paul was so spiritually desperate that he begged God; Paul, the man whom Jesus taught; Paul, the chosen one to bring forth the Gospel to the Gentiles; Paul, the one who had already been blinded by Jesus on the road to Damascus; Paul. the one who mentored young Timothy; Paul, the one who was such a model of faith to all the brand-new-baby Christian churches. He told them this in Acts 14:22: *"Through many tribulations we must enter the kingdom."*

Paul had seen churches tossed like dice and people dying for their faith. These young Christians, whom he was preaching to and traveling to see, were being slain for their faith, and he tells them to be strong. Christ Himself preaches to His disciples in John 15:20: *"If they persecuted me, they will persecute you."* Paul knows persecution is part of the job. Paul is faithful through everything—so faithful that he boasts in the Lord and counts everything loss except for knowing His Savior:

> *But whatever things were gain to me, those things I have counted as loss for the sake of Christ. More than that, I count all things to be loss in view of the surpassing value of knowing Christ Jesus my Lord, for whom I have suffered the loss of all things, and count them but rubbish so that I may gain Christ, and may be found in Him, not having a righteousness of my own derived from the Law, but that which is through faith in Christ, the righteousness which comes from God on the basis of faith, that I may know Him and the power of His resurrection and the fellowship of His sufferings, being conformed to His death; in order that I may attain to the resurrection from the dead. Not that I have already obtained it or have already become perfect, but I press on so that I may lay hold of that for which also I was laid hold of by Christ Jesus. Brethren, I do not regard myself as having laid hold of it yet; but one thing I do: forgetting what lies behind and reaching forward to what lies ahead, I press on toward the goal for the prize of the upward call of God in Christ Jesus.*
>
> – Philippians 3:7-14

We know Paul is beaten, stoned, shipwrecked, jailed, and without food and shelter at times, and on top of all that, God gives him a nagging thorn that will never go away. On top of all that He has chosen for Paul to face and suffer, God makes Paul suffer daily with this thorn. By now Paul should be like a spiritual car running only on fumes, but Paul always has a full tank. He is a spiritual boss. He is empowered by His weakness because He knows God gets the glory. God has the strength through Paul's weakness. Paul has a defining endurance that never stops ticking, like a loyal grandfather clock in the entrance hall of a grandmother's farmhouse—like the pendulum swaying back and forth, never to stop.

As women with chronic diseases or disabilities, we can relate. I have sobbed my eyes out on my bed, beseeching the Lord to take my thorn, to take my disease. I have found myself laid out on the floor of my bedroom, thirsty for the water of relief from this disease, broken beyond repair, at times. I've ached so much my throat has the feeling of a carpet burn, and my rib cage so sore from my chest's heaving, unrequited, and uneven breaths that it feels like a caveman has used his club to beat his prey over and over. With tears of my soul pouring-out through my bloodshot eyes, I've recounted all the times I've lost out and not been part of so many wonderful, cherished memories with my husband, daughter, family, and friends. Like you, I bear horrific pain and suffering with my thorn, and when I go to bed at night, I pray that God would take it, but if He doesn't, that I would be content, be a witness through it, and find my peace in the awesome works of His will. It is well with my soul! You are not alone, my friend. I encourage you to brave through your emotions, gathering your heart back up, and have faith, knowing He is good. Know you can endure.

SAVING SAUL SPIRITUALLY

When God saved Saul, the young Pharisee was on the road to Damascus, set on his drive to persecute and kill Christians. He had no heartbeat yet for Christ, no conviction, no sanity. He was a monster; a smart, educated, pharisaical brute; a killer for the cause of his Roman country. Christ blinded him and called to him:

> *Now Saul, still breathing threats and murder against the disciples of the Lord, went to the high priest, and asked for letters from him to the synagogues at Damascus, so that if he found any belonging to the Way, both men and women, he might bring them bound to Jerusalem. As he was traveling, it happened that he was approaching Damascus, and suddenly a light from heaven flashed around him; and he fell to the ground and heard a voice saying to him, "Saul, Saul, why are you persecuting Me?" And he said, "Who are You, Lord?" And He said, "I am Jesus whom you are persecuting . . . "*
>
> – Acts 9:1-5

God took a wretched, spiritually blind man and physically blinded him. Paul was physically blinded before Christ just as we are spiritually blinded before Christ. But God's call to both Paul and to us—unsaved as we once were—is permanent. When He calls us, we come. Paul lost his physical sight for a while but gained his spiritual eyes from the Wonderful Counselor. After his sight was restored, he went with Christ Himself to be taught, and Paul was never to be the same. When his learning was complete, the man of God now named Paul was to lead a revolution. His mission? To save the Gentiles. God had extended His grace and the gift of Christ, the Savior, to the Gentiles, and Paul was the man who would lead their conversion. Paul's persecution began right after God's teaching time with him ended. Paul said this about his ministry:

> *Are they servants of Christ? —I speak as if insane—I more so; in far more labors, in far more imprisonments, beaten times without number, often in danger of death. Five times I received from the Jews thirty-nine lashes. Three times I was beaten with rods, once I was stoned, three times I was shipwrecked, a night and a day I have spent in the deep. I have been on frequent journeys, in dangers from rivers,*

dangers from robbers, dangers from my countrymen, dangers from the Gentiles, dangers in the city, dangers in the wilderness, dangers on the sea, dangers among false brethren; I have been in labor and hardship, through many sleepless nights, in hunger and thirst, often without food, in cold and exposure. Apart from such external things, there is the daily pressure on me of concern for all the churches. Who is weak without my being weak? Who is led into sin without my intense concern.

– 2 Corinthians 11:23-29

Yes, Paul endures through desperate hardship, and he has no one at times except His loving God—and that is all he needs. Paul is a saint to whom we with disease can relate. He tows the line; he walks the walk and talks the talk; he is like the president of a company who runs his business with successful endurance and then tells us his secret:

For I have learned to be content in whatever circumstances I am in. I know how to get along with humble means, and I also know how to live in prosperity; in any and every circumstance I have learned the secret of being filled and going hungry, both of having abundance and suffering need. I can do all things through Him who strengthens me. Nevertheless, you have done well to share with me in my affliction.

– Philippians 4:11-13

CONTENTMENT

We learn new things every day while battling disease, and one thing we should make sure to learn, to designate as a key ingredient in our trial-filled life, is contentment. Paul has to learn to be content. He does not wake up one morning magically able to withstand all the mass persecution, the agonizing days in jail, the stoning and shipwrecks. No, believing sisters, we must find our fight, our hope, our perseverance and endurance in learning how to be content, whether living in plenty or living in want. Every day we can pray for contentment, and we can exercise our minds to think on things that give us that inner peace and serenity. Our situation, our circumstances, do not control our contentment. We must learn like Paul to be content.

Paul goes on to say that his strength in his circumstances comes from the spiritual empowerment we have as children of the Living God, from the spiritual freedom of being content with all things God has for us. Our strength is not to beat the disease physically—praise God if he does that—but we need to be praying for the kind of strength that gives us contentment. We need to be praying for God's will and spiritual strength through His Holy Spirit:

> *. . . we are afflicted in every way, but not crushed; perplexed, but not despairing; persecuted, but not forsaken; struck down, but not destroyed; always carrying about in the body the dying of Jesus, so that the life of Jesus also may be manifested in our body. For we who live are constantly being delivered over to death for Jesus' sake, so that the life of Jesus also may be manifested in our mortal flesh.*
>
> – 2 Corinthians 4:8-11

STAY THE COURSE

So, stay the course; stay the path. If you have not yet run to Him, then repent and run to the Imperial Incarnate when He calls your name and let your "old man" die. Die to sin; die to the old person who had no life. You are new, and you have been given Life! You have been called and claimed. Run the race. Sometimes with disease and disability, it's impossible for us to physically accomplish all this. But we can train to be the best spiritual athlete possible, competing not for medals, ribbons, or a first-place, temporal trophy.

Do you remember how important recreational trophies were growing up—whether it was a child's soccer game, a state band competition, a debate team victory, third place in your team's basketball championship, or first place in an all-day, hot and sweaty track meet? We practiced and prepared for the skill to achieve the physical prize, for the physical glory of being the best, many times putting ourselves before others to win first prize. We don't run a race to compete for second place or to let others pass us by; we run for the gold.

The Bible gives us so many examples of competition, but those examples are stressing spiritual discipline, beating up our old habits and ways of living, and equipping ourselves for the glory of the cross, the glory of a beat-up Savior that we should be running to embrace. We should want to win the prize that will strengthen our strides, that will keep our endurance justified in the triumphs of grace, that will spur us to hunger for victory through our trials of hardships. When considering our soul's competitions that we're called to win, remember this: people may run marathons, climb mountains, and use their physical skills to their peak potential, but it's all just toil and labor without the Lord our Maker. Do not let disease or disability keep you from competing for the spiritual prize, the prize to which every trophy, ribbon, award, or prestigious plaque cannot even begin to compare; those are just heaps of junk when compared to Christ's secure embrace and a triumphant shout of praise and hallelujah from the chorus of angels singing in Heaven when a Christ-follower is bid home; we, too, will hear and worship with this chorus, and my friend, that will be the ultimate prize. It's the above-all, brighter-than- the-stars light that guides sailors on the night sail, because He is the luminous star, giving us the light of His blazing glory, the Shakina Glory Himself. Run to that prize. It's the prize we want to win, a trophy that means life forever in His eternal home planned for us. You will be casting off your old clothes and putting on a robe of purple like our King, as a winner who beat the trial, a winner who won the reward of seeing others know the Savior, winning the battle of sin once and for all. We are to keep training and competing until we reach the everlasting ever after.

An excellent resource that will walk you through biblical suffering is the book *Trusting God Even When Life Hurts* by Jerry Bridges; it's one I refer to over and over because of the old stenciled-in-our-soul truths found inside. These truths cannot be erased; they're like a fossil imprint on an old limestone rock. They will stay with your soul and can be wonderful counsel when you're needing a breather, a pick me up, along with answers to tough questions on why mankind suffers.

MORE LOVE TO THEE, OH CHRIST

You are not alone. Today, people across the world are being persecuted and enduring suffering. Here is an account that should be like a memory in motion for you. Use it and recall it when the pain and feelings of defeat are stronger than your will to endure your disease for Christ:

For years, North Korean Pastor Kim and 27 of his flock of Korean saints were living in hand-dug tunnels beneath the earth. But then, as the Communists were building a road, they discovered the Christians living underground. The officials brought them out before a crowd of 30,000 in the village of Gok San for a public trail and execution.

They were told, "Deny Christ, or you will die." But they refused. At this point, the head Communist officer ordered four children from the group seized and had them prepared for hanging. With ropes tied around the children's small necks, the officer again commanded the parents to deny Christ. Not one of the believers would deny their faith. The parents told their children, "We will soon see you in heaven." The children died quietly. The officer then called for a steamroller to be brought in. He forced the Christians to lie on the ground in its path. As its engine revved, they were given one last chance to recant their faith in Jesus. Again, they refused. As the steamroller began to inch forward, the Christians began to sing a song they had often sung together. As their bones and bodies were crushed under the pressure of the massive rollers, their lips uttered the words:

"More love to thee, O Christ, more love to Thee
Thee alone I see, more love to Thee
Let sorrow do its work, more love to Thee
Then shall my latest breath whisper Thy praise
This be the parting cry my heart shall raise
More love, O Christ, to Thee."

Never did any of these martyrs deny their Lord but were faithful to Him to the end. Throughout history, people of faith have sung during their last moments on earth. To the astonishment of their tormentors, they have joyfully raised their voices in praise to God. They have counted their life as rubbish. How? How in such great torture and pain have the saints been able to endure? We know how to suffer like this; we can suffer righteously because of the good days ahead for us. The gates are open that take us into the kingdom of our own Suffering Lord. These Christian martyrs knew they would obtain a better resurrection. They were looking to what is unseen. In the words concerning Abraham, they were looking to a heavenly home. A.W. Pink, a renowned Bible teacher, says this:

"Let it be remembered that they were men and women of like passion with us: their bodies were made of the same tender and sensitive flesh as ours are, but such was the care they had for their souls, so genuine was their faith and hope in a better resurrection, that they listened not to the appeals and whinings of the outward man."

– A.W. Pink[7]

I long to be with God in eternity, and when I read about these believing saints, it gives me the courage and the understanding to face my suffering and to sing jubilantly:

"More love to thee, O Christ, more love to Thee
Thee alone I see, more love to Thee
Let sorrow do its work, more love to Thee."

My husband said this in his Sunday school class as he was teaching:

"In the vice grips of affliction as the mortal man is squeezed, outpours from faith a clear and pure testimony."

I will endure because I belong to a God who has been gracious. Yes, I will suffer. But my dear husband captured it perfectly. Can you continue to suffer in Christ, trusting Him with your quotidian affliction? Believing sister, we understand God allows suffering, but we can endure, and we can trust in Him and His ways. Before we go any further, we need to talk about where suffering and disease originate and how you came to a have disease or disability from God.

THE BLUE PRINT

God created you for His glory and His purposes.

7 Pink, Arthur W. *Studies in the Scriptures 1934-1935: Volume 7 of 17*. Lafayette: Sovereign Grace Publishers, Inc. 2005.

" . . . 'So that the rest of mankind my seek the Lord, and all the Gentiles who are call by my name,' says the Lord, who makes these things known from long ago."
– Acts 15:17-18

If you can start there with the blue print, then everything else can be built on that. Treasured friend, you need to know that you were made by Him and for Him.

"Everyone who is called by My name, and whom I have created for My glory, whom I have formed, even whom I have made . . . "
– Isaiah 43:7

Before time in eternity past, God created you. Every part of you. From your height, weight, color of skin and hair, to your gender and every outside physical characteristic, all was given to you by the Sovereign Ruler who designed you exactly the way He purposed for you.

"Know that the Lord Himself is God; it is He who has made us, and not we ourselves; we are His people and the sheep of His pasture."
– Psalm 100:3

When You think about this, you should be in constant awe that He formed you and took time to design and shape you. See these helpful verses:

And even the very hairs of your head are all numbered.
– Matthew 10:30

The LORD said to him, "Who gave human beings their mouths? Who makes them deaf or mute? Who gives them sight or makes them blind? Is it not I, the Lord?"
– Exodus 4:11

See what great love the Father has lavished on us, that we should be called children of God! And that is what we are! The reason the world does not know us is that it did not know him.

– 1 John 3:1

Just as He made you on the outside, He also fashioned you on the inside. Each heartbeat, the connecting of your bones, the signals from your cells and nerves, your immune system, and the way blood moves through your veins, are all ways He has given you life inside. You are a gorgeous mirrored-but-still-marred reflection of His image . . . and you are here breathing, very much alive. Do not let disease deaden your heart on the inside. This is how you were made; this is how you were created. Since disease is here in this world, it can corrupt bodies, and pain and suffering will continue because man is flawed. He is sinful and without Christ; each has turned to his own way.

"For you were continually straying like sheep, but now you have re-turned to the Shepherd and Guardian of your souls."

– 1 Peter 2:25

Man is corrupt.

"For the one who sows to his own flesh will from the flesh reap cor-ruption, but the one who sows to the Spirit will from the Spirit reap eternal life."

– Galatians 6:8

But in this corrupt world, Christ is our Chronic Redeemer. He pursued and purchased us through His suffering, by His torturous sacrifice of His own life. He is the genuine Breath of Life. He gave you your life; He gives you every breath you take. Spiritually, when you were saved, He gave you the Holy Spirit who pursued you with intensity and who blows where He chooses to blow. He did not have to choose you; He did not have to remove the scales from your eyes, but He did. He pursued the key to unlock the chains that kept you huddled in Satan's dungeon. He is our Pursuer! He has given us the life we are living. It's His gift, even with suffering, and you can live a full life to Christ's glory.

WE'RE SUBJECT TO DISEASE

God does everything perfectly, but because of the Fall of mankind, sin, death, disease, war, famine, suffering, pain, heartache, and sadness all entered the world. In the beginning when God created the world, He created Adam and Eve, the first human beings on earth, and they chose to disobey God. Adam and Eve willfully chose sin over perfect communion and fellowship with Him, and because of Adam and Eve's choice to disobey and rebel against God, He cursed man as well as the ground and earth:

> Then to Adam He said, "Because you have listened to the voice of your wife, and have eaten from the tree about which I commanded you, saying, 'You shall not eat from it'; Cursed is the ground because of you; in toil you will eat of it all the days of your life . . . "
>
> – Genesis 3:17

Now because of their disobedient act, their deliberate and consequential sin against Him, our bodies are subject to disease such as cancer; they are subject to disability, like a child being born with a genetic disorder. Everything in creation is corrupted by the Fall; and everyone is subject to sin—the sin we commit against ourselves, the sin we commit against others, and the sin others commit against us. This means that sin, in some instances, can cause our suffering, such as when a driver under the influence of alcohol hits your car and you are left paralyzed. Our bodies are also subject to natural disasters and being affected by those elements like tornadoes, tsunamis, earthquakes, etc. They are affected by the cursed ground, viruses, plagues, and pestilence.

"Both thorns and thistles it shall grow for you; and you will eat the plants of the field."

– Genesis 3:18

Because the earth was shunned, and Adam and Eve sinned, they were removed from the garden:

Then the LORD God said, "Behold, the man has become like one of us, knowing good and evil; and now, he might stretch out his hand, and take also from the tree of life, and eat, and live forever"— therefore the LORD God sent him out from the garden of Eden, to cultivate the ground from which he was taken. So He drove the man out; and at the east of the garden of Eden He stationed the cherubim and the flaming sword which turned every direction to guard the way to the tree of life.

– Genesis 3:22-24

Man's bodies are subject to disease or disability if God orchestrates it because of His sovereign purposes. The One who stretches out the Heavens like a tent curtain may allow our bodies to suffer the effects of the Fall, but He promises if we are His that He will sustain us spiritually through our trial:

. . . seeing that His divine power has granted to us everything pertaining to life and godliness, through the true knowledge of Him who called us by His own glory and excellence. For by these He has granted to us His precious and magnificent promises, so that by

*them you may become partakers of the divine nature, having es-
caped the corruption that is in the world by lust.*
                                                – 2 Peter 1:3-4

But sweet friend, the Lord also causes great pain and suffering because it's His will and work—to show the beauty of His creation, to show His power, to further the name of Christ. Look at *John 9:1-3: As He passed by, He saw a man blind from birth. And His disciples asked Him, "Rabbi, who sinned, this man or his parents, that he would be born blind?" Jesus answered, "It was* neither *that* this man sinned, nor his parents; but *it was* so that the works of God might be displayed in him."

The works of God are being displayed in your life as well. He has chosen you, my friend, to display His power in your sick body if you are living for Him.

"Whom God will use greatly, He will hurt deeply."
                                                – A.W. Tozer

"God never allows pain without a purpose."
                                                – Jerry Bridges

Perpetual illness is more than hard; it can swallow our very lives and keep us locked up, as a shut-in at home, incapacitated in a bed with soft sheets that now feel like rough sandpaper. Our shelter and heartfelt dwelling is no longer our "home sweet home" but something we want to escape. We want to run away on vacation and come back no longer sick. We feel as if we need a retreat sometimes, but there is none to have unless we know the Rock of Refuge.

*"Incline Your ear to me, rescue me quickly; be to me a rock
of strength, a stronghold to save me."*
— Psalm 31:2

The Lord is my heart's strength and forever portion.
*"My flesh and my heart may fail, but God is the strength of my
heart and my portion forever."*
— Psalm 73:26

Comfort, abundant life, and joy are not found in a physical ability, in visible abodes, on tropical or restful furloughs, or even through being healed, but are found in spiritual birth. Disease can take your body and can remove it little by little or all at once, but it can never take your soul if you have placed your faith in the Lord Jesus Christ. The physical clarity of knowing you hurt terribly in your condition may be with you 'til you die; doctors may never find the right antidote, but as a Christian woman who's been purchased and pardoned by the One who climbed the hill on Calvary's mount, you are alive spiritually. Disease may overtake your flesh, but your soul is guarded and cannot be stolen by the enemy. We suffer with hope; we suffer, knowing God's purposes and ways are higher than ours. We know we cannot search out His ways, but we do know with confidence that our suffering will lead to our "home sweet home" in Heaven one fine day.

*"Great is our Lord and abundant in strength; His understanding
is infinite."*
— Psalm 147:5

SUSTAINED IN THE TRUTH

Friends, no matter what ails you physically, when the day is long and fraught with attempts to cope, and the night is even worse . . .

remember that our loving Christ gives you a supernatural faith and hope that only He can give; and He will get you through the suffering. I know His Word is true; I know His love and His promises will sustain me. I know He will sustain me moment by moment, day by day—just as He will sustain you.

> *"So do not worry about tomorrow; for tomorrow will care for it-*
> *self. Each day has enough trouble of its own."*
> – Matthew 6:34

We must have the faith the size of a mustard seed—faith that says we believe in Him for salvation and are willing to trust Him with our disease, that we're willing to pursue righteousness and holiness. No, we're not perfect yet; we are touched with sin.

HIDE IT UNDER A BUSHEL? NO!

Suffering with a cyclic physical disease, disability, or condition is a moment by moment, minute by minute, hour by hour, day by day, week, month, year, never-ending calendar of trials. A fixed disease or disability affects our life, keeping us at times from family, friends, social gatherings, and even our church. It's debilitating, and it suffocates the soul when the pain comes in droves, like a steam truck lowering its head and plowing over your bones and pummeling your desire to see the Truth. Your soul can only cry out for God's mercy, that His will be done and not your own. Disease or disability can keep you from church when you so desperately want to go, when you want to see your child performing in the choir or fulfill your turn in bringing snacks in Sunday school. You've missed seeing dear friends, there's a new believer's baptism, and more than anything, your heart needs the corporate worship and the teaching that will strengthen you by God's Word.

Yet, your condition doesn't take a break to let you catch your breath. It doesn't let up but persists and grows stronger and stronger, like an infection that wants to spoil your soul and become gangrene. It's life on fast forward with no remote control to stop the lingering disease you're undergoing physically and spiritually.

When we endure suffering, we know we're not alone. But our responsibility, our truest devotion and heart's desire, should be to please our Lord and Savior while we're here on this earth. Regardless of the circumstances we face, we are called to be disciples, witnesses, and lights for Him. Our light cannot be hidden under a bushel. We cannot let our pain and disease bombard our thoughts and security in the promise of the scriptures and the work of the Holy Spirit in our lives. We are called to be righteous. We have a good and faithful Savior who suffered with us, and we have the example of Job.

JOB, THE RIGHTEOUS

If you remember, I talked briefly about Job at the beginning of the book. The story of Job leaves me breathless and humbled to my knees when I think about all he encounters. It keeps things in perspective for me; Job is like no other man. He is righteous, and God tests his faith, He tests his strength, and He refines him without Job ever knowing why he suffers in the first place. Job not only suffers with physical pain in his body, but with oozing sores and enflamed boils. He suffers through an unthinkable trial: the loss of his home, livestock, and children. Job is left to sit in a heap of ashes wearing torn sackcloth, using rocks' sharp points to scratch his pitiful skin. Job suffers in the heap of mocking accusations from his friends and wife; in fact, she tells him to curse God and die. Job struggles with doubt, and then

Job does something he can never take back: he questions God. When God speaks back, it's through the storm. "Through the storm" would mean His voice is commanding and His voice booms. The frequency and tone shoots through the torrential downpour—and the storm cowers. God, in fact, is putting Job in his place. Job is reminded he is a lump—a lump of clay—and God is the Potter.

> *Woe to the one who quarrels with his Maker—*
> *An earthenware vessel among the vessels of earth!*
> *Will the clay say to the potter, "What are you doing?"*
> *Or the thing you are making say, "He has no hands?"*
> *Woe to him who says to a father, "What are you begetting?"*
> *Or to a woman, "To what are you giving birth?"*
> *Thus says the Lord, the Holy One of Israel, and his Maker:*
> *"Ask Me about the things to come concerning My sons,*
> *And you shall commit to Me the work of My hands."*
> *– Isaiah 45:9-11*

Job is told to: *"Now gird up your loins like a man, and I will ask you, and you instruct Me!"* (38:3). By the end of the book, God has lambasted Job for trying to question Him. Job can only repent in ashes. Listen to how Job changes his tune, how he is visibly jostled and shaken, slapped in the face, and is now awake in his acknowledgement and recognizes the God of the nations as His Potter:

> *Then Job answered the Lord and said,*
> *"I know that You can do all things,*
> *And that no purpose of Yours can be thwarted.*
> *You asked, 'Who is this that hides counsel without knowledge?'*
> *Therefore I have declared that which I did not understand,*
> *Things too wonderful for me, which I did not know.*
> *Hear, now, and I will speak;*
> *I will ask You, and You instruct me.*

I have heard of You by the hearing of the ear;
But now my eye sees You;
Therefore I retract,
And I repent in dust and ashes."

– Job 42:1-6

Job suffers for God's will to be done, and he repents of his questioning. I have never experienced that degree of loss; I have never lost my home or my income, and to think about losing my daughter and my husband sends a shutter down my spine that immediately makes me numb and lifeless. I know that some of you who are reading this may have suffered horrendous losses of loved ones, and my heart and flesh cry out to the Lord right now on your behalf.

Even though I suffer from disease, I have never had my husband or friends tell me to curse God and die; I am truly humbled by Job. I have learned from this great patriarch, the man more righteous than any other, the one handpicked by God for Satan to tempt . . . who am I to question; where was I when God tamed the Leviathan?

Can you draw out Leviathan with a fishhook?
Or press down his tongue with a cord?
Can you put a rope in his nose
Or pierce his jaw with a hook?
Will he make many supplications to you,
Or will he speak to you soft words?
Will he make a covenant with you?
Will you take him for a servant forever?

– Job 41:1-4

And where was I when God made the Behemoth?

"Behold now, Behemoth, which I made as well as you; he eats grass
like an ox."

– Job 40:15

God was giving Job examples of the power He has over the beasts
He created, the creatures He made. Only God has that supremacy, and
only God is the One I should put my trust in when I'm enduring
unmitigated pain.

We want the first part of the story. We want to be able to gird up
our loins and trust. We don't want to hear His voice from the storm. Job
does not know why he suffers, but as we see in Scripture, the answer
is staring straight at us in one verse . . . Job is righteous:

The Lord said to Satan, "Have you considered My servant Job?
For there is no one like him on the earth, a blameless and upright
man, fearing God and turning away from evil." Then Satan an-
swered the Lord, "Does Job fear God for nothing?"

– Job 1:8-9

Job doesn't know why; his wife doesn't; his friends don't.
Otherwise they would never offer the foolish counsel they do. They
don't know why he suffers, but we do: he is righteous. God puts him
to the test to see if he will score a perfect grade, to see if he can pass
the test of trusting God in the tough times as well as the good. God
has given Job all the earthly desires he wants. He has wealth, livestock,
flourishing land, a family, his health . . . and Satan knows this. He
tells God that Job will always praise Him in the good times, but if
God takes it all away and causes him pain and suffering, he predicts
that Job will curse God. Job doesn't curse God, but he does question
Him, and God refines him in his suffering.

Remember, we are refined through all our pains and loss, and like Job, we can strive to be righteous in our suffering. This is something we can do within the suffering of our disease, in and out of seasons of pain. God teaches us through Job's life. Instead of questioning and letting your heart sulk in misery because of your disease, lift up your head, lift up your hands, and repent if you have questioned God. And then . . . strive to be righteous. God chooses Job to suffer because he is righteous. One reason He chooses us to suffer from disease is to refine us and to help us become righteous.

The definition of "righteous" is blameless and upright.

"The Lord said to Satan, 'Have you considered My servant Job?
For there is no one like him on the earth, a blameless and upright
man, fearing God and turning away from evil'."

– Job 1:8

The holy, righteous God describes a fallen, sinful man as doing no evil in His eyes. Is God calling someone blameless? That's beyond the best compliment you could ever receive. God let those words He said be placed in His Word. God knew that we as believers would read how he describes Job. This is a man who endures his whole life taken away—replaced with death, pain, and insurmountable loss—all in one moment, everything gone. And God knew that Job would recognize that he was but dust and learn through what he encountered—through the conversations with the Lord Himself that God is powerful, mighty in His works, and the world's Owner and Creator; the whole world is His. And God calls Job blameless.

"A man will be justified by faith when, excluded from righteousness of
works, he by faith lays hold of righteousness of Christ, and clothed in
it, appears in the sight of God not as a sinner, but as righteous."

– John Calvin

Job was righteous because he feared the Lord; he had reverence for his Maker. In the Old Testament, everyone was under the Law. They needed animal sacrifices to meet the Law of God's demands.

> *". . . because by the works of the Law no flesh will be justified in His sight; for through the Law comes the knowledge of sin."*
>
> – Romans 3:20

Jews and Greeks were all under sin as Romans 1:18 says: *"The wrath of God is revealed from heaven against all unrighteousness."* But Christ was not yet born and the sacrifice for sin had not been met until that fateful but glorious day that He became the Lamb that takes away the sin of the world. After Christ sacrificed His sinless life on the cross and became the propitiation for our sins, we were no longer under the curse of the Law, but the Law was and is like a tutor that shows us that no one is worthy, and we all fall short.

As John MacArthur explains, our righteousness comes from an alien and foreign righteousness that we cannot or will never be able to attain.

> *"This is the only solution. A righteousness has to come down to us, a righteousness that is alien to us. God has to come Himself to our rescue. God has to give us a righteousness that is outside of us, above us and beyond us. The very one who gave the Law to condemn us must also give the righteousness to save us. This is the light of the glorious gospel of Jesus Christ shining to us. The righteousness that you need and that I need to be saved, Paul says, 'Comes from God, it is the righteousness of God Himself.'"*
>
> – John MacArthur[8]

---

8 "God's Gift of Righteousness." Grace to You, March 22, 2009. https://www.gty.org/library/sermons-library/80-344/gods-gift-of-righteousness.

For us to be righteous, we need only look to the cross, the righteous cross. We are blameless, we are upright, since we were given the righteousness of Christ. We can always be blameless as we endure; we can always be blameless like Job as we endure our own diseases and trials, and like Job, we can humble ourselves and recognize God's omnipotence. Like Job, we will make it through this life, bruised, cracked, but never broken beyond His use.

> *"If the Lord has more witness for you to bear, you will live to bear it. Who*
> *is he that can break the vessel which the Lord intends again to use?"*
> – Charles Spurgeon

You and I will and can endure like Job if we mimic Job's character. We will praise the Lord in the end of our life when we worship anew in mansions of gold, and we can praise Him now as the broken vessels He continues to use.

So why do we suffer? In the next chapter, we're going to learn that suffering has a purpose and offers provision and ultimately protection. Each of these will help you glimpse your disease and suffering through a powerful corrective lens—in a godly view that will make you bold and grateful for His promise.

Remember, in your ongoing suffering, look to others who came before you who suffered righteously: the patriarch Job, the martyred North Korean believers, and Paul the disciple, who just like you had a recurring spur. As seen in each of these examples, the godly suffered yet praised God and counted their life as nothing because they saw Christ as everything.

> *" . . . and upon finding one pearl of great value, he went and sold all*
> *that he had and bought it."*
> – Matthew 13:46

Eternal life is the "pearl of great price," and we should be willing to go through our pain and suffering with bristled endurance, and like the merchant in the parable, sell all we have to purchase it. Suffer righteously; suffer with joyful endurance for Him! More love to Thee, O Christ. Come quickly, Lord Jesus, come!

> "I bear my witness that the worst days I have ever had have turned out to be my best days. And when God has seemed most cruel to me he has then been most kind. If there is anything in this world for which I would bless him more than for anything else it is for pain and affliction. I am sure that in these things the richest tenderest love has been manifested to me. Our Father's wagons rumble most heavily when they are bringing us the richest freight of the bullion of his grace. Love letters from heaven are often sent in the black-edged envelopes. The cloud that is black with horror is big with mercy. Fear not the storm. It brings healing in its wings and when Jesus is with you in the vessel the tempest only hastens the ship to its desired haven."
>
> – Charles H. Spurgeon

Heavenly Father,

Thank You so much that we have never suffered alone—that Christ is our example. Thank You that You are with us always through Your Word, that our endurance comes not from human strength we build up in our own power and might, but that it comes from the death that Christ died and the resurrection He obtained, as He sits at the Father's side. Our weakness and knowing we can do nothing in our own ability, but that it's Christ working in us for His good pleasure, are our strength and our endurance that get us through the pain and suffering of our own chronic disease. Help us to endure with righteousness, like Job; without fear, like the North Korean believers; and with hearts that entrust our pain and disease to You.

Amen!

QUESTIONS:

1. Did God make suffering? Or allow suffering?
2. Where does endurance come from? List a verse.
3. How did Adam and Eve sin? What happened to the earth because they sinned?
4. Why did God create you?
5. What are some reasons for suffering?
6. Did Paul suffer?
7. What did Paul say is the secret to going through trials?
8. What is the definition of righteousness?
9. Who was Job? Did God spare Job's suffering even though he was righteous?
10. What did Job learn because of his trial?
11. Do all diseases or disabilities happen because of sin? What verse assures us that disease or disability is not always because someone sinned?
12. What are you learning because of your trial with disease or disability?
13. How can you be more content? What are some verses that you can meditate on or memorize to help you?

Chapter Seven

THE CHRONIC PURPOSE

"The secret is Christ in me, not me in a different set of circumstances."
– Elisabeth Elliot

But to the degree that you share the sufferings of Christ, keep on rejoicing, so that also at the revelation of His glory you may rejoice with exultation.

– 1 Peter 4:13

My Sister in Suffering,

We learned in the last chapter that God allows suffering because the first man sinned, yet God did not create it. For me, that makes a significant difference in adjusting my mindset, my heavenly perspective, each morning and every day. But I don't stop there; with my thoughts always moving, I think on the next related question: what is suffering's purpose? I like to go all the way back to Creation, when God placed Adam and Eve, the first man and woman, the sinless couple, in the sublime and sacred garden, where He walked and talked with them in the cool of the day. He gave them the key to the front door of every whim and happiness, lasting joy, all their heart's desires; and they wanted for nothing. He created them inadmissibly incomparable, each of them sculpted with His mastery design. They were made only for each other.

Before Eve, Adam was not complete. God gave Adam a stunning crème de la crème like no other, made before time, a stunning bride, exceeding everything Adam could have imagined. After God created the animals, Adam's job was to name each one, and God said it was "good." Then He put Adam into a deep sleep, and He created Eve. For God to make Eve out of Adam's own rib shows the connection, the meaningful glue—like a forever-hopeless, lasting, giddiness-in-the-core-of-your-heart, holy and soul-soothing, loving relationship. And then things were "very good."

"God saw all that He had made, and behold, it was very good. And there was evening and there was morning, the sixth day."
— Genesis 1:31

God, who made you, created the first woman. I can only shake my head and put a halfway grin on my face, with my wide eyes imagining what she looked like. Her physical beauty would have put Hollywood's A list to shame. And remember, she had no makeup, no plastic surgery, no Botox, no facial creams, no home-shopping network's latest exercise thingamajigs to tighten and tone up her aging muscles and skin. Eve, the refreshing beauty, unalloyed, supernaturally and flawlessly made, sheer and utterly honed, was created out of Adam's rib. Can you imagine when he woke up after his long nap and there before him stood the most stunningly attractive woman designed to fit him, and only him: the one and only Gorgeous Eve. The kindness of God to give him a partner only made suitable for him makes me smile; no wonder marriage is so sacred. It's a covenant created by God to bind you with the perfect helper suitable for you.

I could never dream of having anyone other than my literal match-made-in-Heaven, my husband, Brad. God knew who would suit me:

a strong, patient, strong-in-the-Word, mature-beyond-his-years in wisdom and knowledge, godly husband. He gave him to me for so many reasons in this life. I could not be living with this disease without the love of Christ I see in my husband every moment of my life. He is the provision God has provided for me, and God provides for you as well, through the means He uses. A friend, a doctor, your church, a godly mentor, your spouse, your family, a neighbor, and supernaturally in ways and means we can't even see and begin to understand.

"Consider the ravens: They do not sow or reap, they have no store-room or barn; yet God feeds them. And how much more valuable you are than birds!"

– Luke 12:24

My husband loves me with every speck that is within every fiber of his being. He loves me sacrificially, like Christ loved the church and gave Himself for her.

"Husbands, love your wives, just as Christ also loved the church and gave Himself up for her."

– Ephesians 5:25

I know Brad would lay down his life for me at all cost. He sacrificed so much at such a young age to enter into matrimony. While he was in college taking classes, he was also working nonstop to pay for my wedding ring. He cleaned carpets, gave plasma, and even drove buses. His relationship with the Lord was his top love and priority. Brad at twenty years old had, and to this day will always have, a selfless heart with an old soul. He loved the Puritans, the Reformation, and the theologians from that time period; and so much of who he is comes from the influence of those wise, old teachers and preachers of the

Word in his life. I know he would take this disease from me if he could. He is the most selfless man I've ever met. He is my leader and my once-in-a-lifetime, school-girl-crush-turned-reality love of my life. I used to dream of marrying him when I was a bean-pole, stringy-haired, twelve-year-old little girl, and I remember doodling his last name with my first name. But that's another story for another time.

Brad is perfect for me, and even though Adam and Eve were perfect for each other, they wanted more; they wanted to be like God. Adam and Eve had an unbreakable bond and communion; they walked and talked with God. They enjoyed words shared with their Maker, laughter in the paradise of peace, strolls surrounded by a decadent maze of soaring plant life and a color wheel of fruits and vegetables of every shade and kind; the garden was a farmer's market of delights and pleasures to satisfy their taste buds. Adam and Eve had the divine source of true life and sustenance because they had God Himself. But it wasn't their taste buds that couldn't be satisfied; it was their hearts—their selfishness and "me complex." It was all about them. They wanted their own kingdom, the omnipotent mind of God, and a scepter with which to rule and be like the heavenly-ordained Son who wears the jeweled crown.

We all know the rest of the story. They ate of the forbidden fruit: the bite that caused the evil and dreaded Fall of mankind. The snake's words tricked their tempted hearts, and their sin brought about the Fall and opened the deadly floodgate of sin.

"Through one transgression there resulted condemnation to all men."
– Romans 5:18

The battering ram was unleashed, breaking our hearts and capturing us, taking us away as its slave, a slave of sin. Any sin causes some form of suffering, either directly and/or indirectly. God cursed the earth and allowed Satan's oily manipulation and lies to make the once-guiltless couple experience shame and embarrassment. They realized their nakedness and vulnerable exposure and then tried to cover themselves with the plants and leaves they once saw growing wild and free. The fig leaves, once a forever green landscape, now served as a hedge of manual protection for their bare skin. The pride of self-love proved too much, and they surrendered the umbrella of protection God offered them; they hid in shame after their lips tasted the only food He commanded them not to eat:

> They heard the sound of the LORD God walking in the garden in the cool of the day, and the man and his wife hid themselves from the presence of the Lord God among the trees of the garden. Then the LORD God called to the man, and said to him, "Where are you?" He said, "I heard the sound of You in the garden, and I was afraid because I was naked; so I hid myself." And He said, "Who told you that you were naked? Have you eaten from the tree of which I commanded you not to eat?" The man said, "The woman whom You gave to be with me, she gave me from the tree, and I ate."
>
> – Genesis 3:8-12

Man was forced out of the garden, never to return. Now without the Father caring for them, with no more tender talks as they strolled in the tranquil and divine oasis, man now had to labor and live off the ground, and God cursed the ground as well:

> Both thorns and thistles it shall grow for you;
> And you will eat the plants of the field;
> By the sweat of your face
> You will eat bread,
> 'Til you return to the ground,
> Because from it you were taken;

For you are dust,
And to dust you shall return.
– Genesis 3:18-19

Not only did Adam and Eve suffer by having to now work the corrupted ground, but all women, beginning with Eve and every woman after, would now suffer physical, often excruciating pain during childbirth.
"To the woman He said, 'I will greatly multiply your pain in child-
birth, in pain you will bring forth children; Yet your desire will be
for your husband, and he will rule over you.'"
– Genesis 3:16

Decaying earth and physical pain were now reality because of Adam and Eve's choices.

Our bodies also suffer because our outward man is decaying due to living in a fallen world.
"Therefore, we do not lose heart, but though our outer man is decay-
ing, yet our inner man is being renewed day by day."
– 2 Corinthians 4:16

The first Adam and every man after would now suffer physically—and also spiritually, without communion with Christ. As John MacArthur said, "We inherited the *guilt* of sin, meaning we inherited the *corruption* of sin."
"... through the one man's disobedience the many were made sinners."
– Romans 8:19

No one is innocent; no one is pardoned. We're all born sinful. By Adam and Eve's choice to willfully disobey the Holy One, sin entered the world. And suffering began.

We know we have suffering because of Adam and Eve's sin. As we learned, sin is breaking God's Law. Adam and Eve were commanded not to eat of the Tree of Knowledge of Good and Evil, yet they chose to disobey and eat. Eve willfully chose her me-complex over forever fellowship with God. She preferred her blatant disregard and willing ignorance, her arrogant, unholy, and cursed choice to take in her hand the forbidden fruit. She was the first woman on earth who dared to become like the One who rides the wind and who reigns on High—the One who shaped her, named her, sheltered her, and loved her. Eve was the first woman to know her Spiritual Father, and she vanquished the relationship with one bite. She then handed the fruit over to her husband, enticing him to take a bite, and so he did. Sin was birthed and then permeated the earth and the heart of Adam and Eve. Sin not only consumed them but has been passed down from generation to generation; we inherited the sin from the first man:

> Therefore, just as through one man sin entered into the world, and death through sin, and so death spread to all men, because all sinned—for until the Law sin was in the world, but sin is not imputed when there is no law. Nevertheless, death reigned from Adam until Moses, even over those who had not sinned in the likeness of the offense of Adam, who is a type of Him who was to come.
>
> – Romans 5:12-14

However, we sing Hallelujah for the rest of God's story, the plan of redemption:

> Therefore, having been justified by faith, we have peace with God through our Lord Jesus Christ, through whom also we have obtained our introduction by faith into this

grace in which we stand; and we exult in hope of the glory of God. And not only this, but we also exult in our tribulations, knowing that tribulation brings about perseverance; and perseverance, proven character; and proven character, hope; and hope does not disappoint, because the love of God has been poured out within our hearts through the Holy Spirit who was given to us.

For while we were still helpless, at the right time Christ died for the ungodly. For one will hardly die for a righteous man; though perhaps for the good man someone would dare even to die. But God demonstrates His own love toward us, in that while we were yet sinners, Christ died for us. Much more then, having now been justified by His blood, we shall be saved from the wrath of God through Him. For if while we were enemies we were reconciled to God through the death of His Son, much more, having been reconciled, we shall be saved by His life. And not only this, but we also exult in God through our Lord Jesus Christ, through whom we have now received the reconciliation.

– Romans 5:1-11

SUFFERING HAS A PURPOSE

Just look at how our Savior suffered . . . His body emptied of vitality, His soul and spirit crushed. Christ in all His suffering was dying an inmate's death to set us free, to rescue us, to rescue His rebellious, sinful children from eternal jail, from Hell itself, and from being without our Father. His suffering gave us a relationship with His Father, a relationship we did not deserve or earn. His love for us compelled Him to remain on the cross. He could have called down legions of angels, He could have come down, but He stayed nailed to the wood, His flesh ripping. I cannot imagine the pain of knowing His Father heard him yet looked away, that it pleased Him to crush His Son for all mankind, for me and for you. The spiritual anguish of losing the protection of His Father is like asking me to turn my head when I hear my daughter crying. Instead of looking resolutely away, I rush to her side when she falls, even with the smallest scrape and drop of blood, but not so our Heavenly Father when He let His Son's blood pour out like a raging waterfall, for you and for me.

The purpose of suffering is . . . we are sinners, and we had to die to sin once and for all. Christ gave us salvation and suffered for that purpose, His purpose. The Father gave up Christ for me? I can't even make it one moment without sinning, and yet He chose me. He chose me and you by sacrificing His humanity and defending our souls by surrendering His. By taking on the Fall of humanity, by taking on sin, He saved us from the spiritual death that we should have died. If we understand this, then we know He suffered, too; we're not alone, and we know that Jesus suffered to accomplish the Father's will. Let us suffer to do His will! Let us suffer with purpose. If we must suffer, let us do it the way our Lord modeled it—with trust and hope, with submission and obedience to the Father.

As Christ was dying, He was still using His life to witness. He shared the Truth with the dying thief; He promised him paradise:

One of the criminals who were hanged there was hurling abuse at Him, saying, "Are You not the Christ? Save Yourself and us!" But the other answered, and rebuking him said, "Do you not even fear God, since you are under the same sentence of condemnation? And we indeed are suffering justly, for we are receiving what we deserve for

our deeds; but this man has done nothing wrong." And he was saying,
"Jesus, remember me when You come in Your kingdom!" And He said
to him, "Truly I say to you, today you shall be with Me in Paradise."
– Luke 23:39-43

As we go through our plight of disease, we can still put others' lives before our own in the hope and trust that, as we share the Good News in our infirmity, souls can be saved. Mankind needs the Gospel just as the thief on the cross needed Christ. We can be a disciple with a purpose—our purpose to still share and voice with triumph the message of the cross, the message of crucifixion that saves the hurt, the broken, the cursed, the diseased. Christ gives us His purpose and promise of salvation, and like we learned with Job, we're not to question or grumble but to be as righteous saints, to be those who will suffer as Christ suffered. We must look at suffering and face it straight on, understanding God's purpose, provision, and protection through it, and ultimately, the perfection we will gain through it. We cannot endure physical suffering without understanding our God and His divine Scripture that teaches us suffering's meaning. We must keep our suffering in eternal perspective: He is with us, and He suffered with us.

The sin we committed and the sin we will commit were defeated on the cross. We may still feel disease's ugly tentacles as this world won't be made new like the garden until Christ returns and sets up His kingdom, but the purpose of His suffering ultimately fulfilled God's plan. Christ took our sin, and we have perfection. How great is that! God sees us as spotless, a coheir, and innocent before His eyes. The Holy God of Israel looks on you with His blazing justice and holy eyes and sees you through His gaze as pure and innocent yourself.

That helps me put my disease and the sin I've committed in my flesh in perspective. I'm innocent in the holy, reverent eyes of Christ. Every sin—past, present and future—He does not see if we are His. He looks at us and sees righteousness; He sees Christlikeness.

Friend, we will always have disease and pain because of the Fall, but God did not just leave us after the Fall to keep wallowing in our sin and leading ourselves to damnation. He sent Christ. Christ became sin. We became Holy, blameless and righteous. We became without blemish in His sight. That's God's purpose: to send Christ to die and suffer on the cross so that we can have salvation; and to rescue a people to Himself that will put His glory on display. Nothing is ever an accident. He sent Christ on purpose and with that purpose.

Praise God He does all things on purpose and in His purpose. He gives us a foreign, all-spiritual provision and protection that will lead to perfection when you stand before Him at His Bema seat. So, take in the blessings of God's purpose and how He will provide for us, protect and perfect us, with a disease from which we try to run, and know He will give us an escape route.

"No temptation has overtaken you except what is common to man-kind. And God is faithful; he will not let you be tempted beyond what you can bear. But when you are tempted, he will also provide a way out so that you can endure it."
– 1 Corinthians 10:13

We don't have to escape or run from our disease, like hurling a frisbee whisked through the air that disappears beyond sight. We need to know God is providing for us, protecting and perfecting us, through all the many trials that come our way.

We need to understand God's provision through the trials of living with a disease or disability, His protection through it, and His perfection one day in Heaven, giving us Life without a diseased body. This should give us hearts that love Him more and are not so apprehensive about our struggle. Praise the Lord He does this for us! He will fill your heart and mind with lively hope and a smile that tells your soul He is looking after you. So, come along with me, and let your soul be free in the stillness of the moment. Know that He is God and know that the God who is mindful of the deer giving birth is mindful of your disease. The God who provided for Joshua as he blasted his horn and the walls came down will give us that same spiritual provision and protection.

CHRIST AS OUR EXAMPLE

When Jesus made His way out into the garden the night He was betrayed, He took His closest disciples for comfort and support. He wanted them with Him. He was about to give up His life, and He was innocent. I can imagine the scene as Christ is slowly and sorrowfully pacing in the garden, about to offer up the prayer that could change the course of humanity, that could save Him from torture and crucifixion, that could save him from the taunting crowds, mocking and spitting on him, that could save Him from separation from His Father, the tears and sweat turning to blood; He pleaded, *"My Father, if it is possible, let this cup pass from Me;"* but then added, *"Yet not as I will, but as You will"* (Matthew 26:39). We should always be selfless in our suffering and look at our Jesus and His example.

I know the temptation to want my own way as I suffer with disease, and that's why I think often about Christ in the Garden of Gethsemane.

At times I want my will, my way, for "this cup to pass from me." I want physical healing, and I want it over God's will. I can identify with Peter, who denied Christ three times:

> Now Peter was sitting outside in the courtyard, and a servant-girl came to him and said, "You too were with Jesus the Galilean." But he denied it before them all, saying, "I do not know what you are talking about." When he had gone out to the gateway, another servant-girl saw him and said to those who were there, "This man was with Jesus of Nazareth." And again he denied it with an oath, "I do not know the man." A little later the bystanders came up and said to Peter, "Surely you too are one of them; for even the way you talk gives you away." Then he began to curse and swear, "I do not know the man!" And immediately a rooster crowed. And Peter remembered the word which Jesus had said, "Before a rooster crows, you will deny Me three times." And he went out and wept bitterly.
> – Matthew 26:69-75

I deny my Savior when I choose my way, my sin. But our delightful Father, the Source of unchangeable light, my God in His magnificent and immeasurable grace, my Refuge to the end of times, always forgives me when I think those thoughts, when I act bitterly. With a repentant heart, I come to Him in prayer and ask for forgiveness, for renewal and refreshment from His Spirit once more. When we suffer because of our disease or disability, it helps to know why, to recount all we go through with spiritual eyes and not the rose-colored glasses of the world.

THE FATHER MAKES US LIKE HIS SON

> "The mortification of the flesh is the quickening of the Spirit."
> – John Calvin

The purpose of suffering is to make you like Christ.
"After you have suffered for a little while, the God of all grace,
who called you to His eternal glory in Christ, will Himself perfect,
confirm, strengthen and establish you."
– 1 Peter 5:10

Our purpose is not just our own as we daily try to imitate Christ, but to brace up under pain and trial, not letting Satan have a foothold on our disease.
"No temptation has overtaken you but such as is common to man;
and God is faithful, who will not allow you to be tempted beyond
what you are able, but with the temptation will provide the way
of escape also, so that you will be able to endure it."
– 1 Corinthians 10:13

Our purpose is to see joy and contentment in where God has us, to trust Him with our disease. I can strive to live with this disease with the hope and promise that He is enough.
"These things I have spoken to you, so that in Me you may have
peace. In the world you have tribulation, but take courage; I have
overcome the world."
– John 16:33

We understand the purpose of suffering when we see it as a means or opportunity for our suffering to lead others to Christ. We can shine like a brand-new copper penny on a sidewalk as we stand out from others who are without daily pain, without disease or disability. We can share the Gospel of Good News with people who see us and think we should be mad, sad, depressed, or angry. We can share with people who think we should hate God because of what He's allowed for us. Instead of looking like the world and cursing

God for the trials that have brought disease or disability into our life, we can look like the Son, knowing He suffered and that His purpose is anchored in His redemptive plan of salvation, to grow like Him. How do we grow like Him? We become spiritually stronger, more progressively sanctified, the more we lean on Him; the more we read His Word, memorize it, and put it into practice; the more we let the work it does in our lives brim over into others like a pitcher of lemonade overpoured and flowing into a glass on a nice summer's day. This is how we represent Christ to others, pouring out our lives, spilling our hearts out as we speak the Gospel. Our joy, our faith, our life in Christ with disease should stream into others' lives, the more we trust Him in our trials. With our pain, with our lives, with the more we share the Gospel, the more we can bring Him glory and make His name known.

So beloved, this is one purpose of suffering; this is how we can outlast our suffering: by looking like Christ and living with that purpose:

> "Christ is not in the heart of a saint as in a sepulchre, as a dead Saviour that does nothing; But as in his temple, one that is alive from the dead. For in the heart where Christ savingly is, there he lives, and exerts Himself after the power of that endless life, that he received at his resurrection. Thus every saint who is the subject of the benefit of Christ's sufferings, is made to know and experience the power of his resurrection."
>
> – Jonathan Edwards

IN GOD WE TRUST

Another purpose of suffering is to deepen our dependence on God alone, not on our own strength or devices, and not with dependence on the world to mature us. The world takes us further and further from Christ, like a kite whose string snaps and is blown, dancing jerkily in the wind, as the open sky swallows it up whole. But we are in the world holding onto Christ, like that small child, white knuckled with sweaty palms, holding onto a kite for dear life, not onto earth's promises of giving us all we want but nothing we need. It's now socially correct and tolerant to accept, heartily agree with, and act in ways that God's Word declares a clear sin. This occurs within a world that hates our God and despises our beliefs. Sweet sisters, I may live on this earth, but I'm not a true citizen of this country. Ultimately, I'm a citizen of Heaven, and my dependence is on Him, not on a generation in which Truth is relative and corrupted. Our world believes there is no God, or that we're each our own God, or that God is whatever you say He is, simply a higher power who I create myself and who wants me only to be happy. We cannot do anything right or true that's independent and without the Lord; we must trust in Him alone.

NEBUCHADNEZZAR

Before Christ, Nebuchadnezzar was pompous, full of himself, a king who ruled by his selfish heart and not the selflessness his people need. He rejected God. In fact, he was his own God. And because of the arrogance of his sin, God caused him to suffer harshly. God took his kingly status and reduced him to a beast; like livestock, he ate grass and lived among the animals. God took him to the lows of despair, and he suffered alone in the wild, thrown outside, and ignored by his kingdom. Night after night, day after day, he lived like that.

THE VISION FULFILLED

All this happened to Nebuchadnezzar the king. Twelve months later he was walking on the roof of the royal palace of Babylon. The king reflected and said, "Is this not Babylon the great, which I myself have built as a royal residence by the might of my power and for the glory of my majesty?" While the word was in the king's mouth, a voice came from heaven, saying, "King Nebuchadnezzar, to you it is declared: sovereignty has been removed from you, and you will be driven away from mankind, and your dwelling place will be with the beasts of the field. You will be given grass to eat like cattle, and seven periods of time will pass over you until you recognize that the Most High is ruler over the realm of mankind and bestows it on whomever He wishes." Immediately the word concerning Nebuchadnezzar was fulfilled; and he was driven away from mankind and began eating grass like cattle, and his body was drenched with the dew of heaven until his hair had grown like eagles' feathers and his nails like birds' claws.

– Daniel 4:28-33

Nebuchadnezzar thought he didn't need God. Look at his response before God made him like the beasts and banished him: *"Is it not by my power and my majesty?"*

Sisters, we do not have power over anything in our lives; we are not ruling on high and being called majestic. There are no angelic beings in the heavens continuing to praise us without ceasing, repeating in harmonious union, *"Holy, Holy, Holy is the Lord God Almighty, who was, and is, and is to come"* (Revelation 4:8). We did not create the earth by speaking it; we do not control the wind, nor cause the rain to fall on the righteous and unrighteous; we did not before time create a plan of redemption for broken mankind; we cannot step in and out of time or breathe and give man a soul; we did not exist before life even existed; we cannot wipe out entire civilizations that ruled the earth with one look, one word; we are not omnipotent, knowing each person's thoughts, all at the same time, and every person's decisions simultaneously; we cannot raise others from the dead, or walk on water, or heal the blind and lame by touching them.

We may think we're independent, our own kings, our own gods, that we can handle the pain, or progression, or the complicated feat this disease has brought, but like Nebuchadnezzar reigning without our God, we see how quickly our own strength causes us to be like Israel, who continued to stiffen their neck, or like Pharaoh, who hardened his heart. We harden our heart by not trusting and depending on Him. Our dependence is on our God who rules on high; we can always depend on Him through the trial of our languishing disease.

God teaches the mighty King Neb that, as earthly impressive as he is, the core of his being can be knocked to the ground to become a beastly creature with claws; and through this story, God wants to teach us that He has all power and all dominion; He is Christ Alone,

and He turns our weakness into strength. He alone commands the armies and gives the victories. God makes nations a drop in the bucket.
"Behold, the nations are like a drop from a bucket, and are regarded as a speck of dust on the scales; Behold, He lifts up the islands like fine dust."
– Isaiah 40:15

He makes the population of people look like tiny grasshoppers at the base of His thundering feet:
*It is He who sits above the circle of the earth,
And its inhabitants are like grasshoppers,
Who stretches out the heavens like a curtain
And spreads them out like a tent to dwell in.*
– Isaiah 40:22

God laughs at His enemies from Heaven.
"He who sits in the heavens laughs, the Lord scoffs at them."
– Psalm 2:4

He is the One who makes the heart like a flowing stream, following where the Lord is leading.
*"The king's heart is like channels of water in the hand of the Lord;
He turns it wherever He wishes."*
– Proverbs 21:1

He is the Lord of Hosts. He is the Commander of the Angelic armies, giving out orders in the heavenlies to protect us from the enemies' darts. Depending on ourselves to understand suffering and disease is like saying we're a black belt in karate when we can't even kick. We cannot listen to man's views or depend on what we think, such as turning to self-help books, psychiatrists, advice from worldly counselors, our own emotions, or our own fortitude to try and skim through life by the skin of our teeth. *"My bone clings to my skin and my flesh, and I have escaped only* by the skin of my teeth" (Job 19:20).

Like Job, Nebuchadnezzar is trying to escape death and knows he just barely made it. Barely making it without Christ does not equate to making it with Christ; we're to do the opposite of "barely escaping" but, instead, sell out to utter dependence, assurance, reliance, and trust, as Nebuchadnezzar finally does:

> But at the end of that period, I, Nebuchadnezzar,
> raised my eyes toward heaven and my reason returned
> to me, and I blessed the Most High and praised and
> honored Him who lives forever;
> For His dominion is an everlasting dominion,
> And His kingdom endures from generation to generation.
> All the inhabitants of the earth are accounted as nothing,
> But He does according to His will in the host of heaven
> And among the inhabitants of earth;
> And no one can ward off His hand
> Or say to Him, "What have You done?"
> – Daniel 4:34-35

When Nebuchadnezzar becomes beast-like and roams in the wilderness instead of climbing palace staircases and walking marble halls, when he is no longer waited on hand and foot but lives away from the plush comfort of having all and needing nothing, when his life is no longer purposed in earthly majesty, layered in false idols and self-worship, but he lives among the wild beasts, God is showing him he is just a powerless, small, little king. God alone is powerful, worthy of praise, and even as He causes suffering, He is our Warrior

Lion—our awesome King whose home is in Heaven and who causes the mountains to quake and tremble:

The fool has said in his heart, "There is no God."
They are corrupt, they have committed abominable deeds;
There is no one who does good.
The Lord has looked down from heaven upon the sons of men
To see if there are any who understand,
Who seek after God.
They have all turned aside, together they have become corrupt;
There is no one who does good, not even one.
Do all the workers of wickedness not know,
Who eat up my people as they eat bread,
And do not call upon the Lord?
There they are in great dread,
For God is with the righteous generation.
You would put to shame the counsel of the afflicted,
But the Lord is his refuge.
Oh, that the salvation of Israel would come out of Zion!
When the Lord restores His captive people,
Jacob will rejoice, Israel will be glad.

– Psalm 14

Our awesome God cares about the sparrow. Our awesome God restored Nebuchadnezzar when he gave God the glory and recognized that He is the king over all the inhabitants of the earth:

Let the glory of the Lord endure forever;
Let the Lord be glad in His works;
He looks at the earth, and it trembles;
He touches the mountains, and they smoke.
I will sing to the Lord as long as I live;
I will sing praise to my God while I have my being.
Let my meditation be pleasing to Him;
As for me, I shall be glad in the Lord.

Let sinners be consumed from the earth
And let the wicked be no more.
Bless the Lord, O my soul.
Praise the Lord!

– Psalm 104:31-35

We depend on Him for our life and breath. We depend on Him to give us the power to call out His name and pray His will be done, even if that means facing excruciating hurts. In adversity and agony, our dependence on Him deepens our trust in Him as He refines us. We can trust God and depend on Him to help us through our suffering; we can see it not as life through the eyes of the once-kingly Nebuchadnezzar who roamed the land as a beast of burden, but instead like a child dependent on a Father who cares—a Father who gives us every good and perfect gift. *"Every good thing given and every perfect gift is from above, coming down from the Father of lights, with whom there is no variation or shifting shadow"* (James 1:17).

HIS PURPOSE CULTIVATES DEEP ROOTS

The second thing we need to know and embed in our souls is that God made you for His purposes and His glory, and He made you on purpose just as you are. When Job is being tested by all his losses, each devastating and unimaginable, including the loss of all his children, his home, his financial security, and his health—when he is struck with disease, trying to understand why he's in such a large amount of pain and why he must endure it, wondering if it will ever end—we can understand. At times we relate because we don't understand our disease or disability and why we suffer as well. We can relate to Job.

During all this suffering, God tells Job that He is the Potter and Job is the clay—no answer needed. God's plans should warrant trust and obedience as well as our pursuit to be Holy as we go through them. Job suffered so much pain, both physical and emotional as he lost his children, but he never once cursed God. He made you and me just like Job, whether we're sick or healthy, whatever our skin color, whether we're a mom or daughter, a teenager or grandmother, married or single, homeschooled, Ivy League educated, rich or poor, a new believer or seasoned in spiritual maturity. We're all called to make Him shine like a spotlight so that the magnificent radiance of His glory is put on display. It's put on display not only in our lives but like a Broadway stage, with floodlight beams arcing down, not just for the lead cast but for all the audience, supporting cast, stage hands, and crew. You're on point with everyone, so be bright! Be bright like the angels who blinded the sky and shared the Good News with the shepherds on a lonely, pitch black night, announcing the birth of the Messiah! If we have stage one cancer or stage four; if we're terminal or cured; if we suffer pain that crackles like the embers in a fire, with nerves that zing like pin pricks, with a body that's crippled and knotted like an old oak tree, with fatigue that never sleeps . . . even then we are alive in Christ. Know, my friend, that Hope is alive! Bring Him glory! Keep your city on a hill ever shining:

> *You are the light of the world. A city set on a hill cannot be hidden; nor does anyone light a lamp and put it under a basket, but on the lampstand, and it gives light to all who are in the house. Let your light shine before men in such a way that they may see your good works and glorify your Father who is in heaven.*
>
> – Matthew 5:14-16

Be that city as the verse describes, and as you go through disease, trust Him that the embers of His glory will glow as you externally magnify who He is to others. Just like clay that must have a potter wielding and forming it, giving it shape, so are we in God's hands, shaped, created, and made on purpose. As He shapes us, His thumbs pushing, imprinting, stretching, and compressing our clay body, it feels like we're a Christian Gumby, being worked over into a piece ready to be burned in the kiln. Like a gimpy tree with toothpick-thin branches, weak and unable to even hold up a bird who wants to perch, He refines and prunes us. It's beyond laborious, beyond harrowing, but that pruning will only produce fervid, lush leaves on a resilient and sturdy branch. We need to be pruned to have deep, cemented roots for Christ. Disease or disability, even with its incomprehensible pain, with its symptoms and side effects from medicine and blood work, with its physical exhaustion and emotional sorrow, will only make us deep-rooted—with the roots He's given us submerged deep in soil. When we're soaked with more trials and face persecution, when our physical body is in disarray and our emotions want to win, the spiritually stronger we become; and the more He prunes, the more we look and act like our Savior. Our faith can withstand. We can be the godly woman who trusts in the Word, the godly woman with disease or disability whose faith is blooming from a healthy tree, making us every day more like Christ.

He will be like a tree firmly planted by streams of water,
Which yields its fruit in its season
And its leaf does not wither;
And in whatever he does, he prospers.

– Psalm 1:3

These are all purposes of God bringing disease into our lives, for God allowing suffering in the world. Suffering is because Adam and Eve sinned, and the world and man have been subject to the Fall. The world is stained dark, and the ruler of the world is behind every evil act and everything not built on the Word:

> *And you were dead in your trespasses and sins, in which you formerly walked according to the course of this world, according to the prince of the power of the air, of the spirit that is now working in the sons of disobedience. Among them we too all formerly lived in the lusts of our flesh, indulging the desires of the flesh and of the mind, and were by nature children of wrath, even as the rest. But God, being rich in mercy, because of His great love with which He loved us, even when we were dead in our transgressions, made us alive together with Christ (by grace you have been saved).*
>
> – Ephesians 2:1-5

But God can use anything for our good. Suffering is not snobby or cliquish. It can affect anyone; it has no preference: a newborn, your aging grandmother, your high school sweetheart turned faithful husband, your daughter just starting her high school sophomore year, your son just celebrating his tenth birthday, your best friend since childhood, a precious niece or nephew, family members you see only in pictures from your once-a-year family reunion, your enemy you need to make peace with, your Christian brother and sister, your Mormon neighbor just diagnosed with breast cancer . . . and even you.

Disease and disability infest and infect all the world; they show no mercy. But our hope, our joy, rests in Christ's promise. If you are in Christ, your earthly tent is just a shell. We are one day perfected in Him without suffering; He chose for us to be purposed for His use, with the Love and plan He had for us to walk through while we "walk by faith and not by sight."

I'd like to summarize this chapter with one of my favorite Scripture passages, one I've memorized and say over and over when I'm really suffering:

> *For we know that if the earthly tent which is our house is torn down, we have a building from God, a house not made with hands, eternal in the heavens. For indeed in this house we groan, longing to be clothed with our dwelling from heaven, inasmuch as we, having put it on, will not be found naked. For indeed while we are in this tent, we groan, being burdened, because we do not want to be unclothed but to be clothed, so that what is mortal will be swallowed up by life. Now He who prepared us for this very purpose is God, who gave to us the Spirit as a pledge.*
>
> *Therefore, being always of good courage, and knowing that while we are at home in the body we are absent from the Lord—for we walk by faith, not by sight—we are of good courage, I say, and prefer rather to be absent from the body and to be at home with the Lord. Therefore, we also have as our ambition, whether at home or absent, to be pleasing to Him. For we must all appear before the judgment seat of Christ, so that each one may be recompensed for his deeds in the body, according to what he has done, whether good or bad.*
>
> – 2 Corinthians 5:1-10

Memorizing these words and keeping them close to your heart will bring your focus back to Christ and not what you're experiencing in that moment, or in the rest of the moments of your day. Think on the Spirit being your pledge, the seal of salvation; think on having a strong faith; think on Christ loving you and making you like Him though these trials, and how you can serve others as you yourself are walking through your pain. Remember the purposes of suffering. Remember that we are temporal but will one day be eternal! Praise God! Come quickly, Lord Jesus, come!

Precious Lord,

Thank You so much for the ultimate purpose of suffering: that Jesus is the reason, and I am a child of God whom You have redeemed for Yourself and for Your glory. Thank You that I am made with purpose and on purpose. Please help me to think on Your truths and Your love for me when I'm feeling daily anguish from my disease or disability. Thank You that I put my trust in You, God. Thank You that I can use the trial You have given me to be a light for Christ and the Gospel. Thank You, Lord, that this life is temporal, but life with You is eternal.

Amen!

QUESTIONS:

1. What is the ultimate purpose of suffering?
2. What are two more reasons for suffering we talked about in this chapter?
3. Why did God make you? How did He make you? Were you made on purpose or by accident?
4. How can God use you with your disease or disability?
5. What is one of your favorite verses in this chapter? Why?
6. Commit to learning or memorizing 2 Corinthians 5:1-10 if you can. If not, just look over it when you need encouragement. What verse in this passage really encourages you? Why?

Chapter Eight

CHRONIC PROVISION AND PROTECTION

"We cannot trace God's hand, but we can always trust God's heart."
– Charles H. Spurgeon

You, O Lord, rule forever; your throne is from generation to generation.
– Lamentations 5:19

Strong Sisters,

In our world today we have burly, powerhouse countries that flex their muscles with massive military prowess, thinking they control the world like putty in their hands. But no military or government institution, no king, czar, or dictator, no atomic bomb or fighter plane loaded with missiles, can overtake our God who destroyed sin and who reigns over Heaven and earth.

"The Lord will reign forever, your God, O Zion, to all generations. Praise the Lord!"
– Psalm 146:10

Our God is over all.

We live in a world instituted by Him, not by man, and the Lord through His Word has called us as believers to submit to government. *"Every person is to be in subjection to the governing authorities. For there is no authority except from God, and those which exist are established by God"* (Romans 13:1).

America is a free country built on those who fight and protect for liberty, for justice, and for the word "freedom" to actually mean we are free. People serve our government and risk their own safety every day to put our lives first, and we as Christians are called to do the same.

> *"Beloved, let us love one another, for love is from God; and everyone who loves is born of God and knows God. The one who does not love does not know God, for God is love."*
>
> – 1 John 4:7-8

Men and women fighting wars and battles across the globe have seen their blood soak the ground with the color of cherry red pride, bravery, and love for the people they died protecting. But their abilities to protect and defend are still finite and limited because we serve a divine Defender whose power and might is inconceivable. *"It is He who made the earth by His power, who established the world by His wisdom; and by His understanding He has stretched out the heavens"* (Jeremiah 10:12).

Human protection cannot compare to the provisions and protections of our Warrior Lord:

> *The LORD will go forth like a warrior,*
> *He will arouse His zeal like a man of war.*
> *He will utter a shout, yes, He will raise a war cry.*
> *He will prevail against His enemies.*
>
> – Isaiah 42:13

As His children, we are still more safe under Emmanuel's protection and provision—even when in the clutches of the lion's den with Daniel; even on the alter with Isaac; even hanging aside the thief on the cross; even when toiling as a slave to the Egyptians or living as a persecuted Christian in New Testament times; and even when serving as a missionary in a country rife with Christian persecution and killing. Our safeguard is stronger than a steel-framed storm shelter, military bunker, or the President's most qualified top-secret agents and bodyguards. God is the One controlling each day we live; He is over everything, and He is our power.

"Yours, O Lord, is the greatness and the power and the glory and the victory and the majesty, indeed everything that is in the heavens and the earth; Yours is the dominion, O Lord, and You exalt Yourself as head over all."

– 1 Chronicles 29:11

As women with disease or disability, our hope, shelter, and mainstay are in the Lord. We do not depend on man: he is flawed. We don't put anything above our dependence and trust in the Lord. We don't secure our stay in man and his cures, in his answers to "Will I get better?" We don't depend on the might of man or on the idols of protection we've built up in our hearts, convincing ourselves to rely only on the possible protection and provision for our health in the finding of a cure, new breakthrough medicines, or a surgeon flown in from across the world boasting the skill and precision of a sought-after celebrity dressmaker. But instead, we rely on God.

We do not put our sole trust in a new drug just approved by the FDA, or even in going to the best cancer center, hopeful their treatment will cure us and set us free from this body of disease. But we wholly and without omission put our protection and provision in God's will to do what's best for us, and for His glory. We can choose with our heart and soul to unconditionally put God's will over our dreams and desires. He calls us to trust and believe—to be strong in His strengthening and might. *"Finally, be strong in the Lord and in the strength of His might"* (Ephesians 6:10).

We know we have Heaven awaiting us, and that through His Holy Spirit, God will give us all we need spiritually to remain steadfast in Him, to battle sin in our trials, as we take hold of His promises:

> *No temptation has overtaken you but such as is common to man;*
> *and God is faithful, who will not allow you to be tempted beyond*
> *what you are able, but with the temptation will provide the way of*
> *escape also, so that you will be able to endure it.*
> – 1 Corinthians 10:13

Through prayer and His Word, He will give us the strength to keep our minds and our trust focused on His character, on His good for us. *" . . . rejoicing in hope, persevering in tribulation, devoted to prayer . . . "* (Romans 12:12).

He will give us the desires of our hearts if our desires are His, which is God's best, God's will and plan. *"Delight yourself in the Lord; and He will give you the desires of your heart"* (Psalm 37:4).

No matter the cost of our suffering, it's nothing compared to the weight of Glory that is ours. *"For I consider that the sufferings of this present time are not worthy to be compared with the glory that is to be revealed to us"* (Romans 8:18).

Our suffering is nothing compared with seeing the kingdom flourish and others brought in to be with us in eternity. *"For God did not send the Son into the world to judge the world, but that the world might be saved through Him"* (John 3:17).

Why are we in fear? Glory is waiting for us on the other side. Why do we fear death in this life?

When I am afraid,
I will put my trust in You.
In God, whose word I praise,
In God I have put my trust;
I shall not be afraid.
What can mere man do to me?

– Psalm 56:3-4

He has proven over and over that He is our Provider and our Protector:
But let all who take refuge in You be glad,
Let them ever sing for joy;
And may You shelter them,
That those who love Your name may exult in You.

– Psalm 5:11

GOD'S PLAN

What we need to understand is that we are provided for and protected even with disease. When man dies, it's because before time it was God's plan and will, His timing, His control. *"Many plans are in a man's heart, but the counsel of the Lord will stand"* (Proverbs 19:21).

Ultimately, we do not die from diseases; we die because, as believers in Christ, God has finally called us Home from this wicked and evil world. This is not our home! We don't need to attach ourselves to the pleasures that only give us monetary comfort. Having terminal cancer that takes over your body, having dangerous brain surgery, being in a near fatal car wreck and in ICU on life support, watching your infant baby undergo major heart surgery to repair a valve, finding out no cure exists for a chronic disease, that you'll continue to waste away . . . these are all unthinkable. These catastrophic realities make us grief-stricken, numb, with emotions like we've never felt before, without words to describe, fighting for air because we feel we can't breathe, and praying for help, mercy, assurance, peace, and healing—and clutching onto the dire hope that God will provide and protect. During these times, we can try to control and fix life, fix the person we love, fix ourselves in our own power, trying to use our own strength.

We can't . . . but we *can* lift our hands in prayer to our Maker and present our requests with all thanksgiving. *"Be anxious for nothing, but in everything by prayer and supplication with thanksgiving let your requests be made known to God"* (Philippians 4:6).

We know that He will protect and provide, but that provision may look different than what we prayed for:

> *. . . but just as it is written,*
> *"Things which eye has not seen and ear has not heard,*
> *And which have not entered the heart of man,*
> *All that God has prepared for those who love Him."*
> – 1 Corinthians 2:9

He may heal us completely by taking us out of this fallen and fleeting world to give us our new Home in Heaven, or He may heal us on earth through the means He has provided, such as through our doctor's care, or He may *not* heal us as we endure our disease much longer on earth, and those are certainly the hidden mysteries, the secret things. *"The secret things belong to the Lord our God, but the things revealed belong to us and to our sons forever, that we may observe all the words of this law"* (Deuteronomy 29:29). They are the mysteries of God we will understand when we pass out of this life and see our Living Hope before us.

PROOF IN SCRIPTURE

In the book of Micah, God is talking to Israel and listing His case against them. He gives them examples of how He has rescued them over and over. His case is against them, and He has recorded the message in the Bible, so we can read it and learn from the sins of their past and know we can trust Him to provide and protect.

Look at what He says:

> Hear now what the Lord is saying,
> "Arise, plead your case before the mountains,
> And let the hills hear your voice.
> Listen, you mountains, to the indictment of the Lord,
> And you enduring foundations of the earth,
> Because the Lord has a case against His people;
> Even with Israel He will dispute.
> My people, what have I done to you,
> And how have I wearied you? Answer Me.
> Indeed, I brought you up from the land of Egypt
> And ransomed you from the house of slavery,
> And I sent before you Moses, Aaron and Miriam.
> My people, remember now
> What Balak king of Moab counseled
> And what Balaam son of Beor answered him,
> And from Shittim to Gilgal,
> So that you might know the righteous acts of the Lord."
> – Micah 1:1-5

The Lord took care of Israel, but they still doubted Him. They doubted after seeing the Red Sea part, the miracle of the "pillar of smoke by day and fire by night," manna raining down from Heaven to feed them, and all the plagues and wonderful, disastrous miracles that God brought upon Egypt through His chosen man, Moses. He sent the plagues as warnings, destroying the people's health and land, even sending the angel of death and taking their first-born son. He tells them to remember these things, so they may know the Lord's righteous acts. We need to remember who He is what He's done, and this verse reminds us of His righteous provision. He took care of His people then, and He cares for us now. They should never have doubted His power and who He is, and neither shall we.

God is an ever forged, pressing-forward General who takes us into battle with only Himself against tens of thousands of soldiers, chariots, bombs, and ammunition—and we are still the victor if we cast off fear of who He is and put our hope in Him. As a fighting General, He's already won the fight for your soul, and even if the fight with your disease rages on, we don't have to fear this world; He is the One who has saved us, and when we're battling for our life and health, fighting our fleshly lusts, etc., any victory we have on this earth is because of Him. The victory has already been won for you on the cross!

These are just a few of my favorite verses on protection and provision. My two absolute favorites are Psalm 121 and Psalm 91. Look over the list, and it will encourage you to read these and pray these, knowing God hears:

- Psalm 144:1
- Psalm 3:1-8
- Psalm 5:11
- Psalm 12:5
- Psalm 34:19
- Psalm 57:1
- Psalm 59:1
- Psalm 140:4

- Psalm 121
- Psalm 91

PSALM 139

This Psalm of David about God's omnipresence and omnipotence is one I read, rehearse, and replay repeatedly to myself, meditating on each word when I am suffering. Because He made me and knows me, I know He loves me and helps me as I suffer. David knew suffering all too well as he was being chased in a murderous rage by a man he loved as a father and by the people he had nurtured, smiled upon, and made an oath in allegiance to protect. David had to run from the people he cherished. He had to escape from friends who were now enemies as they turned on him and tried to hunt him down like a fox for sport. He suffered but not without hope, just as we do. He depended on the Lord to keep him safe, even in the dark of the cave and on the run, being pursued by evil.

"To be right with God often means to be in trouble with men."
– A.W. Tozer

David needed God's protection, a situation in human eyes that would have seemed impossible for him to escape death. As David crouched low, in the musty and lurid cave his faith never waned. His prayers were personal to all he was enduring, just as your prayers are, and he cried out in prayer for provision, protection, and deliverance from his enemies. The blackness of the cave kept David safe, so much so that he could actually touch Saul's robe without him knowing; he was guarded by the Lord. When as believers we have God's protection, we don't need human hands to come to our rescue unless God Himself in His plan for your life providentially provides them. God's protection spiritually is all we truly need when we find ourselves huddled away as the disease keeps hunting us and closing in. This is where God's provision comes in. David declares this provision in his beloved Psalm:

O Lord, you have searched me and known me.
You know when I sit down and when I rise;
You understand my thought from afar.
You scrutinize my path and my lying down,
And are intimately acquainted with all my ways.
Even before there is a word on my tongue,
Behold, O Lord, you know it all.
You have enclosed me behind and before,
And laid Your hand upon me.
Such knowledge is too wonderful for me;
It is too high, I cannot attain to it.
Where can I go from Your Spirit?
Or where can I flee from Your presence?
If I ascend to heaven, you are there;
If I make my bed in Sheol, behold, you are there.
If I take the wings of the dawn,
If I dwell in the remotest part of the sea,
Even there Your hand will lead me,
And Your right hand will lay hold of me.
If I say, "Surely the darkness will overwhelm me,
And the light around me will be night,"
Even the darkness is not dark to You,
And the night is as bright as the day.
Darkness and light are alike to You.
For You formed my inward parts;
You wove me in my mother's womb.
I will give thanks to You, for I am fearfully and wonderfully made;
Wonderful are Your works,
And my soul knows it very well.

My frame was not hidden from You,
When I was made in secret,
And skillfully wrought in the depths of the earth;
Your eyes have seen my unformed substance;
And in Your book, were all written
The days that were ordained for me,
When yet there was not one of them.

– Psalm 139:1-16

Take great comfort in knowing that as David suffered, he was still being shielded, provided for, and protected by the Almighty. We, too, are provided for. We can read this psalm and know He wrote our names in the book ordaining our days. He knows when we rise, and He knows all our ways. You cannot go anywhere He is not. You cannot hide away or run from His Spirit, nor will darkness ever overtake you. The psalm says His right hand will be holding you. He is always with you, and when you are suffering physically and spiritually, know that His light overtakes the darkness, just as David says. Just as David knew.

Friends, sometimes we feel alone and terrified like David, hiding not in a cave from people but from the reality of disease. We feel stomped on, sucked bone-thin and dry, and at times we're like a punching bag—beat up, black and blue, doubting God's provision in this suffering. This psalm shows us just how overwhelming are His love and grace, just how ever-present He is always in our lives. Even before we were born, His love and protection are so evident toward us. Through this psalm, we are assured of and grateful for His love and protection toward those of us with disease, seeing His fence around our hearts to keep out the assailant:

> *I will give thanks to You,*
> *for I am fearfully and wonderfully made;*
> *Wonderful are Your works,*
> *And my soul knows it very well.*
>
> – Psalm 139:14

David knew in his soul that God made him, and just as David was fearfully and wonderfully made, so are you! God doesn't say to David that those without disease or disability are the only ones made fearfully and wonderfully. No, *you* were made wonderfully; God is speaking to you, too! You were made in wonder and delight. David was suffering, but he knew God's Truth—that God was for him and that He would provide:

> *You have enclosed me behind and before,*
> *And laid Your hand upon me.*
> *Such knowledge is too wonderful for me;*
> *It is too high, I cannot attain to it.*
>
> – Psalm 139:5-6

David knew God was keeping him safe, that He was behind him and before him, enclosing him in provision and protection. God does that for us, too. We do not physically feel Him, but we can feel our "new man" being transformed daily if we're trusting in Him, depending on Him, and reading His Word.

Cherished sisters, it's a great and hopeful reminder to us that when we do suffer—whether it be bodily or whether our hearts are severed in pain and sadness because of disease—our Cornerstone has given us provision through His death, momentarily here on earth and, ultimately, perfection in eternity. Just as He provided shelter and peace for David, He provides all things we need physically: our daily bread. *"... Give us this day our daily bread"* (Matthew 6:11).

Jesus included this promise as He was teaching the disciples how to pray through the Lord's Prayer. And more importantly still, He will provide all things spiritually we need as well.

You are no different than David to our God. He loves us all the same, and He will provide for each of His children. To me, it's an astonishing comfort that the same love and spiritual provision given to godly men and women in the Bible—such as Paul, David, Mary the mother of Jesus, John the Baptist, and even Christ the Son—He gives to us; He gives that same love and spiritual provision. My disease does not forfeit His provision. He is the Great Provider. Be exalted, oh God, above the heavens! My provision is my salvation. Disease can never hunt you down, follow you into a cave, or pilfer your eternal future; it can never steal your life spiritually and take away your salvation. Your salvation is God's provision if you are the Lord's.

OUR PURPOSE, OUR PROTECTION, OUR PROVISION, PERFECTION

Great is the Lord and mighty to save! As we learned in the previous chapter, He is our Purpose. He is also our Protection, He is our Provision, and eternally, we will have perfection. No more sin; no more disease. When we are finally raptured disease free to the Promised Land, the empyrean bosom, our bright and never-ending worshipful dwelling, we will see the Father's perfection to us as He clothes us in our perfect and glorified body. *"Beloved, now we are children of God, and it has not appeared as yet what we will be. We know that*

when He appears, we will be like Him, because we will see Him just as He
is" (1 John 3:2).

> *For our citizenship is in heaven, from which also we eagerly wait*
> *for a Savior, the Lord Jesus Christ; who will transform the body of*
> *our humble state into conformity with the body of His glory, by*
> *the exertion of the power that He has even to subject all things*
> *to Himself.*
>
> *– Philippians 3:20-21*

Sweet sisters, long for and know perfection is waiting. Drill it into your head and heart, and keep going, keeping your beliefs secure in the One who knows you have disease or disability and will perfect you in eternity. This should give us hearts that love Him more, with less apprehension in our struggle. Praise the Lord, He does this for us! He will fill your heart and mind with lively hope and a smile that tells your soul you're being cared for, so come along with me and let your soul be free in the stillness of the moment. Know that He is God and know that the God who is mindful of the deer giving birth is mindful of your disease. He gives us a mysteriously wonderful, fully spiritual provision and protection that will lead to perfection when you stand before his Bema seat to have placed on your head the Crown of Life.

> *"Blessed is a man who perseveres under trial; for once he has been ap-*
> *proved, he will receive the crown of life which the Lord has promised*
> *to those who love Him."*
>
> *– James 1:12*

So, take in the blessings of God's purpose and how He will provide for us, protecting and perfecting us with a disease that we try to run from to escape. Perfection is the prize we run for, the pearl we search for, the treasure in a field we sell all for. Perfection is where our mansions are built and will be waiting for us.

"Then the King will say to those on His right, 'Come, you who are blessed of My Father, inherit the kingdom prepared for you from the foundation of the world' . . . "

– Matthew 25:34

And perfection is where our glorified bodies will be. Wrap that around your heart like you're snuggled in a winter blanket on a cold, black night. We will have perfection, but remember, God did not promise perfection here on this earth. In fact, He told us we would have struggles, death, disease, and persecution, that we would be hated by those who hate Christ.

"If the world hates you, you know that it has hated Me before it hated you."

– John 15:18

As a believing sister, take a deep breath and just imagine: when we finally reach the pearly, white gates and we meet our perfection, our perfect God, all this imperfection will be no more. No more imperfect worship, earth, medicine, life—or an imperfect body.

Do not fear your disease or disability; do not fear what man can do to you; do not fear what the world can do. *"These things I have spoken to you, so that in Me you may have peace. In the world you have tribulation, but take courage; I have overcome the world"* (John 16:33).

The God of the Bible sees you right now and is watching, protecting and providing for you in ways you may never see. He is with your child in ICU as she fights for her life; He is with you as you reach the last dose of chemo offered by the doctors; He is with you daily with the disease or disability that is chronic. With a disease that is terminal, He is with you.

You are safer with God as your Savior in the last moments of an exhausting, pain-filled life of suffering, as the beeping monitor slows and then records a flatline, than you are without salvation but rich, healthy, problem-free, and enjoying a carefree life. Eternity for those without Christ is the contradiction of "carefree"; they will be the ones with physical and emotional pain forever. Remember, you have the ultimate protection and provision in Christ, who died and gave you spiritual life, then ever having all the military might and physical, powerful amenities on this earth at your disposal. Having a cure to an epidemic sweeping the world but not the spiritual protection you have in knowing Christ proves a fatal cure.

The world will burn up one day, and everyone will meet her Maker when the Lord determines but understand this: if you suffer even for the rest of your life, it pales in comparison to a life eternal with no more pain and no more disease, a perfected life with a perfect Savior, in the perfection of His Holiness. Heaven is waiting! Your perfection is waiting! Praise God! Come quickly, Lord Jesus, come!

I will lift up my eyes to the mountains;
From where shall my help come?
My help comes from the Lord,
Who made heaven and earth.
He will not allow your foot to slip;
He who keeps you will not slumber.
Behold, He who keeps Israel
Will neither slumber nor sleep.
The Lord is your keeper;
The Lord is your shade on your right hand.
The sun will not smite you by day,

Nor the moon by night.
The Lord will protect you from all evil;
He will keep your soul.
The Lord will guard your going out and your coming in
From this time forth and forever.

– Psalm 121

Mighty and Perfect God,

Thank You for Your power to give us the protection and provision we need as we suffer on this earth with overwhelming trials in our unrelenting disease or disability. You have given us so many proofs of Your love and care over our lives that we can read about in Your Bible—and we are so thankful. Please help us to trust You as the One who provides the care and provision we need. Please help our hearts when we are weak, when our souls need rest and peace, to find it in Your comfort as a shield about us. Give us the strength and desire to accomplish Your will, to follow Your will. And if it's in Your will for us to continue to suffer for Christ, then let us do it with righteousness, suffering and on display for Your glory and purposes. Let my suffering be for Your purpose and Your glory, Lord! And give me Your strength, Your provision, Your protection and, in the end, let me know Your perfection through it.

Let us continue through the empowerment of Your Holy Spirit to continue to die to ourselves daily and carry the burden of disease with joyful hearts because we know You are protecting our hearts and minds spiritually through it. Thank You that this life is not where we stop, but true perfection will be ours in eternity, and we can hold onto that promise. When we are in pain and suffering, keep our eyes on the Truth of the perfection of our bodies when we meet You in eternity, when we meet You and You make us perfect, without disease and without sin. Until then, give us strength in You to keep facing and enduring our chronic disease or disability.

Amen!

QUESTIONS:

1. What can we remember about the purposes of suffering?
2. How does God provide for us with disease? Does he provide physically and spiritually?
3. How? Look at the prayer Jesus prays in Matthew 6:9-13, the Lord's Prayer. Memorize it.
4. How does God protect us? Does He protect us both physically and spiritually?
5. What is one of your favorite psalms from the list? Meditate on it and memorize it.
6. Does God always heal us physically from disease on this earth?
7. How does God make us perfect? When? What is a verse you learned about having a perfect and glorified body, free from disease? When will this happen?

Chapter Nine

CHRONIC DEPENDENCE ON HIM ALONE, NO OTHER

*"Felt weakness deepens dependence on Christ for strength each day.
The weaker we feel, the harder we lean."*
– J.I. Packer

*It is better to take refuge in the LORD
Than to trust in man.*
—Psalm 118:8

Dear Courageous Friend,

Diagnosed with a disease at the age of twenty-two, I felt like someone had taken my life away, like an identity thief had not only swiped my social security number and credit cards but my heart and soul as well. I was going to have to start all over, erase my former life, and live with my new one. I knew disease would change me inside and out. Throughout the following years, I would suffer immense pain, take medicine daily, gain and lose excessive weight, suffer the side effects of steroids, lose my hair, look and feel different, and be in a wheelchair and unable to walk as my joints would swell like blown-up balloons.

During my disease's bouts and flares, I would be a mom in survival mode for my daughter and rely on my husband to do for her many of the "mom things" I so wanted to do. I couldn't walk upstairs to help her pick out her clothes for school, fix her hair, make her lunches, attend her sporting events, take her to the cool science museum, observe God's flawless handiwork as we skipped through the botanical garden, or sit in the sun together just enjoying the summer breeze and watching the butterflies' magnificent rhythms as they hovered from flower to flower. I couldn't swim with her on a sweltering day, savoring the cool water as we floated on rafts and laughed the day away. I was not the one who tucked her into bed and read her favorite bedtime story. Our family dinner table was a blanket on top of our bed, so we could all eat together as a family, so I could just be there with the two of them. And often two to three days would elapse between times of seeing them as I would be trying to sleep off the severe aching and throbbing behind a shut bedroom door and asking the Lord to take the edge off the pain.

I would pray the fatigue would go so I could at least sit up in bed and touch my daughter's face and smooth back her hair. I would miss her Awana programs at church. I was almost nonexistent as a helper or volunteer at her school. I would fidget as I dialed friends' phone numbers to see if they could bring her home from school, my mind so jumbled I couldn't formulate my thoughts into words, so I could compose an email. I felt indebted to friends for taking care of her, and I felt jealousy and guilt since I couldn't do the fun things their healthy bodies allowed them to do. My wifely duties had fallen by the wayside, dirty dishes piling in the sink, unfolded laundry sitting in baskets, no clean white undershirts tucked neatly in drawers for my husband to wear under his business suits for work, no dinner emerging from the oven.

Instead, my husband was running around like an ant scavenging for food for the winter. We grew accustom to fast food, and exhausted as he was coming home from a full-time job, he would still do the cooking. I wanted so much to look like the person the thief had stolen from me. Physically, I was not the same girl my husband had married, and I would never again be that person I used to be. The life I used to live had ended. Like a bird with a broken wing, thrown out into the gusting, howling wind, trying to fly but unable to survive in nature, damaged and unrepairable, changed, never to soar freely and brave the storms and elements of nature—that was me. I was that bird. Disease had broken my wings, and I now had to rely on something else to fly.

I now had to rely on others to care for me, rely on my God even more, and learn to trust and love Him more than I ever had. Yet, learning to love Him more as a broken bird unable to fly, I'm so thankful I am that bird; I'm so thankful He fractured my wings. It should not have taken disease for me to trust Him more, but it did. It's one of the many blessings that so humbles me. I would lean on family, friends, the church, and most importantly, the love and compassion of my forever love, my adoring husband. As wonderful and irreplaceable as my husband and my daughter are, I'm dependent on my God alone.

IN CHRIST ALONE

You are never alone in your trial and struggle. My dependence and your dependence are on Him alone. Your condition is not dependent on doctors; your disease is not dependent on medicine. God may provide these and use them to carry out His will, but our trust lies not in them but in Him. You're dependent on the Great Physician.

Shadrach, Meshach, and Abednego were thrown into a burning furnace, willing to die, willing to burn alive and feel their skin melt to the bone, willing to suffer torturous pain because, with rejoicing, they knew Heaven awaited. They depended on God and trusted Him because their freedom was spiritual. Our hearts and emotions are not what free us from sin; our hearts caught up in worldly passions lead us to our independence from Him. But when we have joy through the Holy Spirit, He smothers our heart in the Truth of dependence on God alone. We have harmony in our hearts because we serve a dependable God. Shadrach, Meshach, and Abednego had joy and harmony in their hearts. Is your heart in harmony, peace-filled and unified with His? It should be! We are free spiritually; we have freedom from sin and death.

Sometimes when I'm getting ready for a doctor appointment or in the hospital battling a disease symptom, I feel by myself, sad and sullen, like the kid no one wants to sit next to on the bus. I know that no matter how many surgeries I have, new medicines I try, or specialty doctors I see, my hope is not in my prognosis or the medicine's potential effects. We have well-meaning loved ones who want healing for us, but they need to understand that since we're in Christ, we *are* healed. If you are in Christ, you have the healing that most people don't. Living life on this earth healthy but without Christ proves the fatal disease.

But we have Christ! We have His amazing grace. We were but orphans, and we're now adopted and brought in. We were spiritually in the cemetery, under a cold slab, covered in dirt with flesh decaying, epitomizing as Christ would say, "a white washed tomb." Before I trusted in Christ, I was a hypocrite; I was a Pharisee; I was a Saul set on exposing and ridding my life of Christianity. I was ten feet under with no heartbeat. But now, I put my faith in our Lord, Jesus Christ.

And if you've done so as well, we are risen, alive, no longer dead but saved. We're healthier than we will ever be because our true health, our spiritual condition, is anchored in eternal life one day. To have physical health but no salvation is the most fatal and terminal disease of all.

We have friends who want us to "see this holistic doctor" or "buy those herbs" or invest in expensive supplements, and then we have our flesh telling us to wear a popular saying, "YOLO," which means "You Only Live Once," on T-shirts, cards, and rubber bracelets. It's a brash mentality that says, "Live it up today," without worrying about consequences. Buying into this mindset, we can start to neglect our godly responsibilities as a wife, mom, and woman because we can feel sorry for ourselves or use our disease as an excuse. We must know the difference of when we can't do something because we're truly physically unable, or if we're just making excuses, feeling defeated, depressed, angry, or complacent. Only we know our bodies and what we feel we're capable of doing. Don't use your disease as an excuse. You are always capable of giving praise to God in worship and prayer. We are not absent as women with disease; we're responsible for how we respond through our actions. We should want jewels on our mansion in heaven, not feathers in our hat on earth. We should do things that have meaning in eternity and not worry about earthly accomplishments.

If you're like me, maybe sometimes you feel guilty because your disease makes you feel useless, not like a godly woman, as you're able only to lie in bed. God does not value who we are based on our works. We cannot earn a taller mansion with more square-footage in Heaven. We cannot work harder and try to impress Him with our chore charts. If your heart is focused on bringing Him glory and not trying to earn brownie points, then your prayers to Him while lying in bed are just as valued as the pursuits of running the church's women's ministry. Having a disease does not steal our passion for loving Christ and obeying His Word. We can do that when we are well or ill. We can pray while we're running to the store or resting on the couch. We can praise Him and tell others about Him while we're at work or permanently disabled. We can praise Him when climbing a skyscraper mountain or receiving our first chemo treatment. We can praise Him when working in the garden or struggling to use the walker.

We don't have to be physically fit to love our Lord and serve Him. He can give us opportunities to use our gifts and talents as women who live with disease or disability, just as much as He can use the triathlete neighbor who serves as the children's choir director. He can use us sick, well, young, old, broken, fixed, filled with joy, or filled with tears. You are His and called to worship, to be "after His heart" like David was. Love Him with all you have in His Son. Being sick does not disqualify us from the eternal inheritance. We are saved, we are His, and guess what? Our disease makes no difference to Him, so serve Him and love Him in every way you can.

My hope is found in Christ and Christ alone. With or without disease, our hope is always in Christ. This does not mean we're not hopeful in medicine and hopeful for doctors to find a cure; we should do everything we can to live with our disease in a way that pleases the Lord, so fighting disease is a good thing. Living life to the fullest, to the glory of our Creator, is right and good!

TWELVE YEARS OF CHRONIC SUFFERING

When we think about the Bible, its true and inspired words, we need to understand that the people in its pages were real. We forget sometimes as we read the Bible that we're learning about actual people. Our minds start to read God's Word as if we were reading a novel, forgetting that His Word is alive, changing our hearts and minds through the supernatural working of the Holy Spirit. Read the Bible with fresh hearts and open eyes. Read the Bible as what it is: Truth. These people were flesh-and-blood men and women who lived on this earth. They are not characters, fairytales, myths, legends, or folktales; they are real, and when we read God's Word, these men and women should come to life in our minds.

Some of these men and women are only mentioned in the Bible in one circumstance, like the woman who suffers with severe hemorrhaging. But her story is recorded in Matthew 9:20-22, in Mark 5:25-34, and in Luke 8:43-48. God includes her pain and suffering for us to read and relate to in the pages of His Word. Remember, friends, we are not alone in our suffering. This woman is yet another example of excruciating struggle and disease.

The hemorrhaging woman could not be healed by any earthly means. Why is this important? This passage is encouraging because our struggle is not alone and, just like her, our dependence lies in no other than the Savior Himself. She had lived with this for twelve years with no cure. Why is her story included for us? I believe one reason is to show her belief and dependence on the only One who could heal her: she believed in Jesus as God's Son. This woman we hear mentioned only once in each of three Gospels suffered 12 years with physical pain.

And while we don't even know her name, Scripture tells us that she suffered from severe bleeding. In biblical times, this would have made her ceremonially unclean. By being "unclean," she would have been cast out, disowned by family and friends, because she was unable to be spiritually cleansed and participate in worship at the temple. It does not tell us more, but we know that in that era, she didn't have access to today's numerous, modern-day medicines, and she did not get to enjoy the modern-day conveniences that most of us today can afford. She could not make an appointment with a doctor, use ice packs to reduce swelling, climb into a hot bath, take aspirin to relieve a headache, or drive to Walgreens to pick up a prescription to ease her suffering. She could do nothing but live in pain every day. We don't know if she had a husband or a family, but if she did, she was probably shunned. And if she were responsible for being a wife and mother, keeping up with her daily duties and chores, she had to survive and live and prepare food, so she was doing work. She didn't have the weekends to catch up on sleep; she didn't get to ever stop. She lived every day bleeding from hemorrhaging. She had no resource to try and relieve her symptoms.

Christ had been doing many miracles in her town, and when she knew Christ was walking down the street, she was desperate enough to grab hold of God. Seeing Christ in the flesh, she had no manners to ask for help or wait her turn to watch Him pass through the crowd. She was in full measure a desperate woman, hungry for healing. She did not care what anyone thought; she knew her dependence and hope rested on the Savior to alleviate her physical suffering, so she reached out and touched the fringe of His robe. She was hopeful in His power, hopeful He was who He claimed to be and could heal her. She believed and trusted so much that she knew if she can just touch His clothing, her body would finally be clean. And so, she did. And a woman who had been suffering from a hemorrhage for twelve years, came up behind Him and touched the fringe of His cloak; for she was saying to herself, "If I only touch His garment, I will get well." But Jesus turning and seeing her said, "Daughter, take

courage; your faith has made you well." At once the woman was
made well.

– Matthew 9:20-22

True friends, the woman is made well because of her faith, because she believes. Christ tells her to take courage, giving us a real-life story of hope. And note that He calls her "daughter," a very personal term of endearment. He wants us to know that we are loved by Him as His child—and that we, too, can be courageous. God can choose to heal us, but He doesn't have to do so; the crux of this story is that she is dependent on Him alone. When we start to lose hope with trust and dependence on God, and even if earthly cures through a new medicine or a specialty doctor may elude us, even though our physical suffering can seem too much to bear, we need only reach out to our Savior and depend on Him. We know that He will give us the courage to meet any foe.

He gives the twelve-years-suffering woman courage, not scolding her for breaking protocol and grabbing His cloak. He calls her "daughter"! He knows we are desperate, too, and desires for us to turn our eyes to Him, to reach out and grab His robe, to respond to His love for us. Just as He knows it is her before He turns around, He knows us as well. He hears our prayers, and we can depend on His faithfulness and love for us to do what is best for us. Then we will wait with trusting minds and patient hearts, being still before the Lord, knowing His plan and His ways are best.

In our prayers, in our cries for healing, our lives should still model that desperate trust in Him as our only Hope. When we get good news, we celebrate knowing He accomplished what He wanted in our lives for His glory, and when we hear bad news, our attitude and person should not shift. We can depend on Him in the good as well as the bad, secure in our faith no matter the result. He knows the suffering, bleeding woman before He even turns around; He feels her touch His cloak. He knows who we are, too, and He knows what is best for us with our disease. If you get low and sad about the physical pain, know the Son of God has given you your own home with Him in heaven; this is our temporal pain. At times the pain feels like forever, but He says, "Be courageous!" Our life is in His plan—and His plan is good!—so find the good in being dependent on Him alone in all circumstances.

Do not put anything before your dependence on Him. Do not depend first on doctors, or healing, or medicine. If the doctors tell you something devastating, take your pain and prayers to the Lord for strength as you face it. Never lose hope that if God chooses, He can heal you here on earth through medicine or a cure, even by changing the makeup of your body so tumors disappear, blood work returns normal, or cancer goes into remission. He can do anything in His power and will.

Matthew records in Chapter 9 so many examples of healing, so we know Jesus can heal, but He does not use the same means as in Scripture, and today there are no disciples to raise people or perform miracles. Christ is not physically on earth in skin and flesh, as a man walking through our towns, teaching and healing the sick as He does in Matthew 35. There are no modern-day prophets who can touch your body or pray a certain prayer for you; there are no modern-day faith-healers. Jesus was going through all the cities and villages, teaching in their synagogues and proclaiming the Gospel of the kingdom, and healing every kind of disease and sickness. That was then. We know now that, when Christ died and was raised by God, He is now in Heaven, not now physically on earth. Our God is with us in and out of the seasons of disease and suffering, just as He was with the bleeding woman, just as He healed her from hemorrhaging because of her faith, because she trusted in Him alone. Oh, Lord, help us to put all our hope in You. Help us to depend on you with or without physical healing.

Christ is waiting for the appointed time when the Father gives Him the authority to take back the earth with swift retribution and rescue His beloved children, punishing those not His who have caused pain and suffering, who have killed, and who have persecuted God's chosen. He will not only execute justice for us but also rid the world of disease and make us new in body. That's when we'll see Him again. But though He's not physically with us, He is still for us and interceding for us. We can depend on Him. Our dependence should always be in Him and His plan for us.

I ONCE WAS BLIND, BUT NOW I SEE

Matthew 9 also records the incident of the two blind men who believe, depending on Him for healing.

> As Jesus went on from there, two blind men followed Him, crying out, "Have mercy on us, Son of David!" When He entered the house, the blind men came up to Him, and Jesus said to them, "Do you believe that I am able to do this?" They said to Him, "Yes, Lord." Then He touched their eyes, saying, "It shall be done to you according to your faith." And their eyes were opened. And Jesus sternly warned them: "See that no one knows about this!" But they went out and spread the news about Him throughout all that land.
> – Matthew 9:27-31

As these men are crying out for mercy, they know who He is, that He is traveling through their city. They aren't deaf, so they can hear the commotion and jubilation as Christ is healing—as the carpenter from Nazareth changes the physical makeup of men and women all around them, as He heals the paralytic and demon-possessed, releasing them from their bondage. And they have heard of Him before their own healing-day as well. Rumors would have been swirling, the whispers of "the healing man," the supposed prophesied King who was going to rule them with an iron fist as a Hero covering the land, and so they make their way to the house where He is, dependent on Him healing them. Jesus is in there, and they know He can heal disease. When He asks them if they believe He can do it, they say, "Yes, Lord." They call Him "Lord," they recognize Him as their Master, and they are His loyal slaves.

We must know Christ as both our Lord and Master as well. Yes, He's saved us from our sin, but we also need to obey Him as our Lord. Our faith propels us to live our lives, even being sick, with dependence on our Master to be with us spiritually in the misery of our trial. Christ tells the blind men that He healed them because of their faith. We, too, can have faith and be dependent on our God; our pain, our hurts, our tears are not lost, and we are blessed because the Lord is dependable. Yes, friends, He healed the blind men, but their healing came because they had to have a dependable Source. Nothing else would or could give them hope, give them healing, and give them comfort but Christ Himself.

Christ tells the healed men to keep quiet, to not to share their story with anyone, because the word of His healing was spreading, and people were coming to Him only for physical relief, not wanting to hear the Gospel. They wanted the Healing, not the Healer of sin Himself, the Promised One. They did not want Jehovah, the personal name of God. We need to remember that physical healing is not our ultimate desire or prayer, but rather to have God's will and glory displayed in our lives, knowing He can use our trial and disease, not only in our lives but in others' as well. We should look in anticipation and awe at the ripple effect of how He uses our disease or disability to impact others, so pray to Christ and know that we can depend on Him. He is dependable! Whether we're cured or healed, or whether our disease keeps progressing and our pain deepens, we know where our dependence rests. He is our Chronic Dependence!

Christ always cares; you'll always have the Father's sure dependability. You can always depend on Him! When you weep, you can depend on Him; when you hurt, you can depend on Him. When awaiting results as you sit in the doctor's office, flipping through a three-month-old magazine while trying to stay calm and focused . . . when the only thing you hear is the sound of your own breathing, painful, labored, and unabated . . . depend on Him! When you're waiting in the lobby while your child undergoes experimental surgery . . . when your own side effects are worse than the medicine and treatment . . . when the doctors have no answer . . . keep depending on Him!—not on results or cures in place of Him. Ultimately, depend on the care of the Father. When the doctors have given up and you're no longer a patient, feeling like just another number and a burden, and they look at you like it's your fault because they can't figure out why your blood tests keep coming back abnormal, know the trust and love of the Father, who He is and that you can depend on Him. Depend on Him!

Depend on Him—when your spouse is so tired in maintaining a full-time job but keeps putting the children to bed. Depend on Him—when your children ask, "When will you get better, Mom?" and all you can do is pull them tightly to your chest and brush their hair off their uncertain, tear-filled eyes. His ways are good and right and true.

When you miss church and feel sad and helpless, when your spouse has used up all his sick days to take you to the doctor or stay with you in the hospital, still depend on Him and not your own way. And even when your child, husband, or someone you love says goodbye to the world, you can depend on Him to see you through. He is righteous and compassionate, and He knows what you need before you even speak it. Depend always on the Lord. *"For by their own sword they did not possess the land, and their own arm did not save them, but Your right hand and Your arm and the light of Your presence, for You favored them"* (Psalm 44:3).

As our Beloved, He sympathizes with our pain and tears. He says He keeps them in a bottle. *"You have taken account of my wanderings; put my tears in Your bottle. Are they not in Your book?"* (Psalm 56:8).

This verse tells us that each tear we cry is kept close, tight to His chest. He does not let one fall to the ground; He does not forget. He keeps each special, wet hurt, bottled and remembered—each tear shed that sears and stings as it rolls down our cheek; each broken memory that swallows our heart; each thought that dispenses gloom like a cloud, displacing the sun and causing raindrops to collect like dust; each daily cry of emotional and physical pain.

In the times you feel like a statue, unable to break free from your disease and caught in the same life pose, just as the subjects in a photo stay frozen in their frame . . . and in the times you draw your knees up and bawl because you feel like your life is set on auto-pilot, each moment monotonous, as you rewind each day and replay each memory over and over . . . then please know this: your tears wiped away with a tissue and tossed in the trash mean something to Him.

The tears of anguish, loss, and death, the ones shed each time you suffer, the ones you cry each time you feel like sleeping the day away as you scream into your pillow, those tears are gathered and held in His bottle. And when you pray, He sees each tear that flows freely from your eyes, sometimes helping you to open and express your heart, other times shed when you're crying out to Him, doubled over with scourging pain and despair that leaves you limp, unable to form the words know the Holy Spirit will pray with moaning for you. Each tear He keeps like a parent rocking her infant in the silence of night, so close to her chest; this is how He keeps our tears bottled up and pressed to His heart. He cares, He loves us, and we can depend on Him as our Father because we are His child. We never have to doubt that He is dependable. Knowing He has our tears should remind us of the great and bountiful love He has for you and that He cares that you have disease. He made you, and if you are His child, then He will make you like Christ. And He can use your disease to accomplish that!

So, whatever physical, long-suffering disease or disability is plaguing your body, you are not alone; so many others suffer as you do. When you think you're alone, remember to reflect on the Truth that people in the Bible suffered as we do—even the pain of God Himself when He took the form of a bond slave and left Heaven to become our Savior, Jesus Christ, God in the flesh.

> *". . . who, although He existed in the form of God, did not regard equality with God a thing to be grasped, but emptied Himself, taking the form of a bond-servant, and being made in the likeness of men."*
>
> – Philippians 2:6-7

People in the Bible suffered, and people all across the world today suffer: people like your coworker; the school crossing guard; the woman in line in front of you at the grocery store; a neighbor you always wave to but who stays to herself; the child being wheeled into the operating room in another attempt to have the tumor removed; the barista who makes your favorite drink at the coffee shop; the man who always sits two rows in front of you at church; the woman in a third-world country who walks five miles just to get a pitcher of clean water to carry back to her family; your own child . . . we are not alone. This gigantic, populated world is full of people who not only don't know Jesus but are suffering with physical diseases and disabilities.

As sisters in Christ, God is our dependence. He is the One we trust. He is the One we place our faith in. Our dependence lies in the Truth of His character—sovereign and perfect—and before time, He created you and determined your time on earth. Both the hemorrhaging woman and the blind men wanted His healing hand to touch them, believing He was the Son of God. They believed in Him. Do you believe that the Son of God has all control and can heal you if He chooses? Do you depend on Him in sickness and in health? The marriage vows a wife makes to her husband at the alter are a promise before God and witnesses of a holy union. The bride is pledging her love and life to her future husband. We are His bridegroom, and our life should reflect the same words that a bride and groom declare at their wedding. "In sickness and in health," we depend on Him and the Truth of His Scripture.

What should we remember about God's dependability? It is forever, unchangeable, not based on my achievements or accomplishments; it's not based on how well I perform in life, not on if I'm healed from disease or not. I can always depend on Him spiritually. He is what you depend on—no other name can satisfy; no other name can give salvation under the sun! He is our Dependence, our Source of Salvation,

and one day in Heaven, our "Source of a New and Disease-Free Body."
Praise God! Come quickly, Lord Jesus, come!

> *Thus says the* LORD,
> *"Cursed is the man who trusts in mankind*
> *And makes flesh his strength,*
> *And whose heart turns away from the* LORD.
> *For he will be like a bush in the desert*
> *And will not see when prosperity comes,*
> *But will live in stony wastes in the wilderness,*
> *A land of salt without inhabitant.*
> *Blessed is the man who trusts in the Lord*
> *And whose trust is the* LORD.
> *For he will be like a tree planted by the water,*
> *That extends its roots by a stream*
> *And will not fear when the heat comes;*
> *But its leaves will be green,*
> *And it will not be anxious in a year of drought*
> *Nor cease to yield fruit.*
> *The heart is more deceitful than all else*
> *And is desperately sick;*
> *Who can understand it?"*
>
> – Jeremiah 17:5-9

Heavenly Father,

Thank You that our dependence rests solely on You. Thank You that we can depend on You to satisfy us with all You have for us on this earth—whether that includes more trials, physical healing, or a poor prognosis. Keep our dependence on You alone, not on the trials and circumstances of this world or our own fleshly desires. Help us to depend on Your will for our lives. Help us to trust everyday and follow in obedience to Your Word, knowing we'll be physically healed in Heaven. Thank You for salvation, knowing You're a dependable God who gave Your Son for us and for our ultimate healing from sin—including the promise of a disease-free body one day.

Amen!

QUESTIONS:

1. Is God dependable?
2. Should we trust in anything and depend on anything more than Him?
3. Does God know what we need before we even ask?
4. How did He know it was the woman hemorrhaging who touched Him?
5. Did the blind men trust God as their Lord and Savior? What does that mean?
6. Can Jesus physically heal us the same way He did in the Bible? Why not? How does He physically accomplish healing today? What are some ways?
7. Is God dependable even if He doesn't heal us physically? Why?

Chapter Ten

CHRONIC FOREVER

*"Good friends are like stars.
You don't always see them,
but you know that they are always there."*
– Christy Evans

*He will swallow up death for all time,
And the Lord God will wipe tears away from all faces,
And He will remove the reproach of His people from all the earth;
For the Lord has spoken.
And it will be said in that day,
"Behold, this is our God for whom we have waited that He might save us.
This is the Lord for whom we have waited;
Let us rejoice and be glad in His salvation."*
– Isaiah 25:8-9

Dear Forever Friend,

As you read the final chapter, I am honestly so sad to end my time with you, but I am also so filled with joy for your courage and bravery to have made it through this journey with me. I hope this book of stored-up nuggets of Truth, spilled out gut-hurts, and scriptural teachings from the Living Word have changed who you are for good. I hope you know you will always be my Chronic Friend. I will keep you in my heart, and when I have pain or suffering, when I'm at the doctor's office or taking my medicine, when I'm lying in bed at night reading my Bible or having a morning quiet time, when I'm in the hospital and see someone with a disease or disability, I will be thinking of you, my dear friend who hiked this Chronic Journey with me. I pray that, like the native birds, you find yourself now returning from the South. The cold climate of not understanding while living with disease or disability is over, and the chaste season of spring now awaits you.

Please know I love you deeply. I may not know you personally or be able to hear your voice or take your hand to squeeze it gently, and I may not be able to lean in and hug you, but this trial—this deeply embedded and, at times, dark providence that God has given you or your loved one—makes you close family. I don't have to see you to know your pleas to the throne, your gray days that can't find sunshine, your famished heart in need of the Word's nourishment. I know you're out there, and I passionately hope this book has been a direct reflection of my tightly-knitted-crochet love for you. You, my fierce, fighting sister, are the one for whom I bend my knees and bow my head. I pray for you. I pray for your life and your continual, steady walk with the Lord.

Faithful friend, I know disease can deflate your heart at times. I know the suffering you go through yanks, jerks, and pulls your body like matchstick-thin shoelaces ripping through the loops of beaten up sneakers. Disease is like a stainless-steel faucet pouring out water upon you, cold and relentless, and the resulting tears you cry could fill the infinite ocean. I know your prayers to end this trial could fill a best-selling memoir, and your pain from suffering could overwhelm a skilled and strategic army, yet though you feel vastly outwitted and outnumbered, you have no reason to fear disease or tremble at death if you're in Christ. There is no fear in death when we have Christ as our Victor, Christ as our Reward. Death takes us into eternity, either with life and love eternal or with weeping and gnashing of teeth and separation from God. One day we will die, and when we take our last breath, we will either be in Heaven in serene rest or with Satan in eternal torment. As believers, we get to choose to die with knowing Christ as our Lord, our Forever Healer; we will die with confidence in His Truth. As a believer, you choose to live life in the confidence and faith that God is in control and that you can trust Him through the pain. You can choose to live with the choice of goodness and righteousness, being blameless like Christ who chose the Father's will to be done. You can choose to live for the Father, to be content and wait; even with your earth-bound body in the throes of disease or disability, you can say, "Not my will, Lord, but thy will be done."

THE OLD STORY

The old story of your life is filled with ripped pages, marred and stained with pain and loss. Yet your story is no longer written in those dying leaves of old. You are no longer living out those fatigued and frayed chapters because, by coming to Christ, your pages are renewed, already published with a copyright in the Savior. You can slam that old book shut and never open it again. That story is over.

You have a new life, a living story for Christ as His child, as His follower. You're leaving the "old" and rejoicing in the "new," just as the disciples abandoned their former life, some leaving family, fishing boats, and occupations for a better, eternal Hope. We leave this earth when we are called. When You think about this world, all the hurt and sin, the disgust of men without the spiritual, righteous compass of Christ, left on their own to indulge in their flesh, you know you will face persecution as you live your life for Christ. The fleshly sins of murder, sexual immorality, lies, greed, pride, etc., will dominate unbelievers, and we know they will face the judgement seat and will be cut off. If they do not repent and trust in Christ, they will have no more chances, be shown no mercy, and be found guilty, but we in Christ are no longer facing His wrath and judgment.

We can thank God we are no longer the enemies, no longer part of that ill-fated family. Our citizenship, our community, our chosen country, is not on this earth. We are not part of an earthly empire fashioned by hands that rule by selfish hearts and philosophies, which stack the tower of man's carnal mind further and further from the mind of Christ. This world's culture is like a modern-day Tower of Babel, with the worldly acting as their own god and living for themselves. But we are built on His Cornerstone, the staunch foundation of the Church, the body of Christ and His kingdom. We will reside in a never-dimming realm, the bright bliss of the Holy City, the New Jerusalem that awaits us at the end of this Life:

> *And the twelve gates were twelve pearls; each one of the gates*
> *was a single pearl. And the street of the city was pure gold, like*
> *transparent glass.*
> *I saw no temple in it, for the Lord God the Almighty and the Lamb*
> *are its temple. And the city has no need of the sun or of the*
> *moon to shine on it, for the glory of God has illumined it, and its*
> *lamp is the Lamb. The nations will walk by its light, and the kings of*
> *the earth will bring their glory into it. In the daytime (for there will*
> *be no night there) its gates will never be closed . . .*
> – Revelation 21:21-25

When we lose someone in this life and the sting of death makes our soul swell with pain, we become allergic to living for a while;

yet peering out from behind our shroud of grief into the homes and huts and hospitals of our abusive world, we can see that we are not alone. Others are dying, others are hurting with us—mothers crying over a lost child, husbands mourning as they experience the death of a darling wife or precious child, friends seeing family members pass from this life. Third-world countries experience death's blanketing kiss as a normal, everyday occurrence, and no matter which corner of the world you find yourself, we weep and cry the same, tears touching every human being—even our Savior, who wept over the death of those He loved, experiencing heartbreak.

It's okay that you cry; it's okay that you hurt. Each day, I pray it will become a little less, that you will be able to breathe a little easier because God is carrying you and keeping your spirit filled with His supernatural peace. Yes, you will weep, but never without hope if you are a believer. Our God cares so much about our hurt and our pain, and He promises He will wipe away every tear from our eyes. *"And He will wipe away every tear from their eyes; and there will no longer be any death; there will no longer be any mourning, or crying, or pain; the first things have passed away"* (Revelation 21:4).

He cares so much that He writes in the final book of the Bible about the martyrs:
When the Lamb broke the fifth seal, I saw underneath the altar the souls of those who had been slain because of the word of God, and because of the testimony which they had maintained; and they cried out with a loud voice, saying, "How long, O Lord, holy and true, will You refrain from judging and avenging our blood on those who dwell on the earth?"
– Revelation 6:9-10

These brothers and sisters are all from different tribes and tongues; they're children, missionaries, and saints persecuted and slain for their faith. Still today, missionaries are dying unthinkable deaths in front of their children, believers are made public spectacles because the unredeemed hate our Savior; they despise Christians and hate our beliefs. We have ISIS and war and destruction because we worship the name Yahweh. But He tells us in Revelation that as the martyrs cry out for justice, God will be quick to answer; He will come back to retake His own and punish those who denied Him, who chose to live for themselves and be their own gods with sin as their master.

Yet we are called to remain faithful in our love for Yahweh, faithful even though some of us are dying with disease, facing immense pain daily, battling symptoms that are disassembling our bodies piece by piece like a child taking apart a toy. He will abide in you, and you in Him; and as you keep the hope, He is with you, His love sustains you, just as He is with all those battling this life's troubles in His strength. Your pain will one day lead to forever perfection, so stand for Christ in your heart, even if you can't stand physically. Even with a walker, wheelchair, or cane, even needing assistance to sit up, even if paralyzed, we can stand for Christ. He will give us His strength to lean on the Cross as we experience temporary affliction. One day we will be done with the temporal and revel in eternal consolation.

THE FINAL CHAPTER

This is the final chapter. My words and my heart have laid bare for you. I did not want this book to be so emotional that you got swept up in your unbearable pain, forgetting that you have Christ. You have His supreme wisdom and His authoritative and inspired Word always at hand to show you how to live. I do not want you to despair in your journey because I know its hard realities. I walk this road with you daily, filled with pain, hurt, and suffering. But when you close your eyes and ask God to give you His strength in Christ, you can sigh with relief through all the pain, knowing one day when you die and face eternity, you will call Heaven your home if He is truly your Redeemer and Savior, if He is truly the Lord of your life and the Lord of your suffering.

I want to keep my disease in perspective. Some of you right now have lost someone close to you and are persevering only by His comfort and His peace; the supernatural faith you have in Christ is holding you up and carrying you. You know your eternal hope is found only in the death, resurrection, and life of Jesus Christ. We don't have any other hope apart from Him. Perhaps you are grieving deeply through the loss of a loved one; perhaps your child is in unmeasurable pain; perhaps you are dying of cancer or a loved one is suffering from disease; or maybe you are battling the pain of a disability—but wherever you find yourself, God is with you. He is with them. His invisible, invincible arms are with your loved ones, and He is gracious, full of mercy.

Death is inevitable; we all have an appointed time, and every day we celebrate a new day, month, or year, even as our bodies take one more physical step toward death. As we age, as we get older, time does not stop. The hourglass full of sand keeps emptying until we see the final grain fall, and though we may want to turn it over, to live life again, we know it means our time for earthly life must end.

Our time here is given to us by Him; God gives us life in Christ to honor Him and obey Him, to be purposeful with the Gospel, and to use each grain of sand in that hourglass as His servants, His faithful. Heaven will be ours shortly; maybe even today for some. We yearn for this rabid world to be defeated, for Christ to set up His millennial kingdom. We want to be with all the saints who came before, the ones who lived with pain and disease, who are now just as healed as we will be. Pain is just a tick of a clock as it passes the next time marker but living forever is praise and hallelujah with the Clockmaker Himself. He is the One who tipped the hourglass to start its flowing sand, and He is the One who ordains its finish as the final grain seeps through the narrow tube to join all the ones collected.

When the sand is gathered at the bottom, our time on earth complete, we may wish we could do it all over for Him, yet that time is gone and past. When the sand runs out for me, I hope I will be found faithful, not faithless. I hope I stored His commandments in my heart and did not store up earthly treasures. I hope I ran well and did not trample His goodness under my feet. I hope I have left behind a legacy of Christ for those I know, to those I met, to those I love. I hope I did not choose myself, following my own rules and fleshly desires. I hope my daughter sees me as a Proverbs 31 mommy and loves the same Savior I came to know as He set His agape love in my heart. I want others to see that through the washing of the Word that cleansed my soul, my heart, my human-ness, that God gave me new birth, and now I am a new creation in His Risen Son. I hope my husband sees me far above rubies. I hope I use my gifts to advance the Truth in a generation that has bought into the lies that Truth is relative and immorality is moral.

Sister, use your time here even with disease or disability to make His name known, to be bold with each grain that could slip through the cracks; don't waste them. And as the last one flows downward, be ready to see the Bridegroom like the virgins with their lamps full of oil, eager and full of spiritual vigor. Be the change for Christ in your generation; be the one who does not seek a cultural Christ, who does not turn itching ears to false teachers. Be the one who puts on a gentle and quiet spirit, the woman submissive to God who does not ask what He will do for her, does not demand her "me-time" or time to "find herself." But be a missionary using your disease to share the Truth. Christ says, " . . . I will be poured out like a drink offering." So, let your sands be poured out for Him. Do not waste the sands of your life. Earthly time runs out, but Heaven awaits.

I cannot even begin to comprehend what some of you are enduring, to experience the loss of a child or husband, to watch the eyes close for the last time of someone you love, to say an earthly goodbye to someone you weren't ready to see pass from this world—even when knowing they were in Christ, knowing that when their flesh died, their soul soared to the Father's house. He has prepared a place for those who have left this earth, and those spotless souls are now cuddled to His chest, embracing His rest under the shadow of His almighty wings.

I won't try to capture what you are living through with my finite words because there truly are none. I can only cry out for mercy to the God who will hold you up and who will not leave. He will not crush you; He will lift the stone that has smothered your heart and buried you in the rubble of doubt. Do not hide in the shadow of darkness but stand and let the light of His Word give you the warmth of a sunny afternoon. Let your soul rest in the Truth of the Spirit, teaching you to rely on His promise, His love. Embrace His mercy like the sun embraces that final tinge of golden and orange ember before dusk sets in. The comfort you need is God and His Word and everything we have learned about Christ as our Chronic Love:

" . . . and He will wipe away every tear from their eyes; and there will no longer be any death; there will no longer be any mourning, or crying, or pain; the first things have passed away."
And He who sits on the throne said, "Behold, I am making all things new." And He said, "Write, for these words are faithful and true." Then He said to me, "It is done. I am the Alpha and the Omega, the beginning and the end. I will give to the one who thirsts from the spring of the water of life without cost. He who overcomes will inherit these things, and I will be his God and he will be My son. But for the cowardly and unbelieving and abominable and murderers and immoral persons and sorcerers and idolaters and all liars, their part will be in the lake that burns with fire and brimstone, which is the second death."

– Revelation 21:4-8

So please keep this in your heart and remember:

Our <u>Chronic Journey</u> with disease and affliction will fade like the lilies of the field, but He gave us <u>Chronic Salvation</u> because of His <u>Chronic Love.</u>

Remember, God's <u>Chronic Word</u> is all we need. It is living and breathing, our tutor for studying how to live in obedience and joy with our disease. Christ's life is breathed out in the scriptures for us to emulate and imitate.

Remember, He is a <u>Chronic Sovereign</u> God. He is always sovereign, in control of everything. The boat may rock, and your sails may rip in the harsh wind, but He is in control of the wind and the seas, and they obey Him. We never must fear; we never must panic or doubt His control over our disease. He is sovereign.

Remember, though we suffer, we can be the tune of salvation to share the Good News of the Gospel. He is our <u>Chronic Witness</u>.

Remember, Christ suffered. Christ faced <u>Chronic Suffering</u>, and you are never without Him in your own pain and suffering. The cross on which He hung was for you; the blood He shed was for you; the crown of nails He wore was for you; the death He died was for you; and remember, the day He rose was for you. He is with the Father and now sits in Heaven interceding for you. Remember, His suffering through His death is what gave you salvation. Christ died for you!

Remember, His suffering has a <u>Chronic Purpose</u>. First and foremost, God's purpose was to show His glory for all to see as He made mankind and redeems His chosen. As His chosen, bring Him glory even in your disease or disability. Remember, suffering also has a purpose of deepening our dependence on Him. When we suffer, we cling to Him for His mercy, truth, love, and compassion—for His will to be done.

Remember, we have <u>Chronic Provision</u> to eternal life; through His sacrificial provision, He provided the way to the Father. Remember, He also provides for us physically, meeting our daily needs, as well as spiritually through His Word and the Holy Spirit transforming and sanctifying us.

Remember, His <u>Chronic Protection</u> is both physical as He looks after us and spiritual as He keeps the enemy from us; He keeps us from sin as we rely on the Truth of His Scripture to be our light in the dark of this world.

Remember, His purpose, provision, and protection ultimately lead to our <u>Chronic Perfection</u>. Our diseases will be written out of the next chapter of our life—our forever Life. Remember, when we get to Heaven with no more disease or pain or disability, we will have new, glorious bodies. Time will never end, and our forever life will go on. Sister, we will be new one day.

Remember, He is our <u>Chronic Dependence</u>; we can spiritually every day reach out to grasp His cloak by trusting in Him and the plan He has for us.

Remember to hold onto the promise of a <u>Chronic Forever</u>. One day life will never end, with no need for time because we will be perfectly Redeemed and have new bodies—one that will never again be sick or disabled, but in which we will dwell forever in the sweet by and by. Hold fast, hold to His Word, and cling to the Truths that Jesus, our Lord and Savior, gave you through the Gospel; this is our Chronic Truth. This is the beautiful world of salvation in our lives.

May the word "chronic" completely take on its different, fuller meaning to you as you finish this book. He is your Chronic Love. We will all share our own book one day together, the new book of our life, each of us having our own Chronic Story. We will eternally live our lives in Heaven as sisters who finally beat disease and disability, once and for all.

As I say goodbye to you, my sister, I pray that this book gave you some encouragement, peace, assurance, and joy, that hopefully you will look at your disease and your suffering differently. I encourage you to suffer with joy and with trust and hope in Christ, living for Him. Please know I love you and can't wait to dance around the throne with you—whole, redeemed, fully sanctified, glorified and healed! So, the only thing left to say is "to be continued . . . " to the Book of Life where He has written our names. Until the next chapter, my chronic sister! Praise God! Come quickly, Lord Jesus, come!

Oh, God, my Chronic King,

Your rich pleasures I taste spiritually even though my physical body tastes pain and disease. I cannot be snatched from Your grasp, pulled away or plucked from Your hand. I will not be shaken by this long-suffering trial. Physical death has no hold on me for I am held by the Father in spiritual life. My pain afflicts my body but not my soul. I have a rested soul even if I have a restless body. I am a new and flourished creation in Christ, and the rust of sin and my old person have rotted away, back to dust, and in its place lies the birth of new soil. I have truly sprouted with Your baptism; I am alive. Nothing can keep me from You; though disease and death may try, I will only taste Your mercy and drink from Your cup, walk beside You in the calm, break bread with You at the table, worship You without effort and a whole soul, not with diseased flesh in my new body.

The morning sun will shine forevermore, and I will rest in Your soul light. Darkness will not embrace me, pain will not rule me, and Your cross is my breath, my life, my find. I have found peace without worry, rest without misery, and Truth without blemish. You are the Life. You are my Sanctuary of retreat, the Wings that envelop me, the Spirit that comforts me, the Rescuer who shelters me. In this life I taste aches and fatigue; I taste pain and suffering, physical and spiritual; but I will taste Your goodness one day. I will taste everlasting Life one day. Surround me with Your peace; surround me with those agents of mercy, the angels I cannot see but who are battling the enemy; and help me to rest in You. Help me continue to rest as I continue to fight the pain, sin, struggle, suffering, and daily trial of my disease or disability. Help me to rest in the knowledge of Your Son, the counsel of Your Spirit, the Source of salvation. Salvation is the smile of my heart. It is the grin of life to know the Everlasting. That is the taste I will crave each day, even as other things will be offered to me, but I will not taste defeat. I will not taste the deadly reward of sin. I will not taste the pain that wants me to hunger with hopelessness. I will taste Your strength, and it will spur on my heart. Help me, guide me, nourish and replenish me in this temporary life until I taste the full pleasure only You give, until You take me to my forever home and I taste eternal life.

Amen.

For more information about
Brooke Bartz
&
Chronic Love
please visit:

Instagram: @justbrookebartz

For more information about
AMBASSADOR INTERNATIONAL
please visit:

www.ambassador-international.com
Twitter: @AmbassadorIntl
www.facebook.com/AmbassadorIntl

If you enjoyed this book, please consider leaving us a review on
Amazon, Goodreads, or our website.